Patricia Solomon

Sue Baptiste

Editors

Innovations in Rehabilitation Sciences Education

Preparing Leaders for the Future

Patricia Solomon
Sue Baptiste
Editors

Innovations in Rehabilitation Sciences Education

Preparing Leaders for the Future

With 10 Figures and 22 Tables

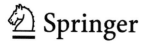

Patricia Solomon
School of Rehabilitation Science
IAHS – Room 437
McMaster University
1400 Main St. W., Hamilton, Ontario L8S 1C7
Canada

Sue Baptiste
School of Rehabilitation Science
IAHS – Room 412
McMaster University
1400 Main St. W., Hamilton, Ontario L8S 1C7
Canada

Library of Congress Control Number: 2005921684

ISBN-10 3-540-25147-2 Springer Berlin Heidelberg New York
ISBN-13 978-3-540-25147-7 Springer Berlin Heidelberg New York

Springer is a part of Springer Science+Business Media
springeronline.com
© Springer-Verlag Berlin Heidelberg 2005
Printed in Germany

The use of general descriptive names, registered names, trademarks, etc. in this publication does not imply, even in the absence of a specific statement, that such names are exempt from the relevant protective laws and regulations and therefore free for general use.

Product liability: the publishers cannot guarantee the accuracy of any information about dosage and application contained in this book. In every individual case the user must check such information by consulting the relevant literature.

Editor: Gabriele Schröder, Heidelberg, Germany
Desk Editor: Irmela Bohn, Heidelberg, Germany
Production: ProEdit GmbH, 69126 Heidelberg, Germany
Cover: Frido Steinen-Broo, EStudio Calamar, Spain
Typesetting: K. Detzner, 67346 Speyer, Germany

Printed on acid-free paper   24/3151 ML   5 4 3 2 1 0

Preface

The genesis of this book arose from our educational consultations with many physiotherapy and occupational therapy colleagues around the world. In the course of presenting workshops that were primarily focused on problem-based learning (PBL), it became very clear to us that educators in the rehabilitation sciences were very interested in other aspects of our curricula. There were questions related to our unique clinical faculty model, our admissions processes, how we incorporate evidence-based practice throughout our programs, and the process by which we develop new models in clinical education, among many others. Physiotherapy and occupational therapy educators were clearly interested in developing creative student-centered learning activities within their own programs. Hence we designed this book to highlight, support, and illustrate educational innovations in the rehabilitation sciences curricula at McMaster University.

Although the Faculty of Health Sciences at McMaster University is known widely as the originator of problem-based learning (PBL), this book is not focused exclusively on this. The intent is not solely to promote PBL, but as its philosophical approach emphasizes student-centered learning and educational process, there are numerous examples and references to PBL throughout the book. Through sharing our experiences with educational innovation we hope to encourage educators to see the importance of integration of content and a self-directed student-centered learning process in developing curricula for current and future practice.

We felt it was important to share the successes and challenges as well as the lessons learned along the way. In doing, so we have tried to incorporate the perspectives and methods used in both curricula. We hoped to model the interprofessional collaboration that we feel is core to health care education and practice. The context and culture of our Faculty is one that encourages an interprofessional approach to education, research, and "being". Thus, another impetus for undertaking the development of this book has been to provide a chance for all of us, as colleagues, to explore our accomplishments together as occupational therapists and physiotherapists. As busy academics, it is all too easy to continue on the path of teaching, research, consultation, service, and administration and not pause long enough to think about the innovations in which we are continually immersed. Writing this book has provided a chance to do just that and to think anew about our challenges and accomplishments.

We also felt it was important to highlight the close collaboration that exists between the occupational therapy and physiotherapy faculty at McMaster University. Although we often approach things quite differently in our separate curricula we have learned much from each other and the debate and sharing that occurs provides a fertile environment for new and creative ideas.

We are most fortunate to be housed in an institution that embraces risk taking and innovation in education. Part of the joy of working at McMaster University is the sense that you will be supported in your efforts to develop new ways of facilitating learning even if these are not always successful.

We are privileged to work with a group of exceptional colleagues who embrace innovation and strive for ongoing excellence in education. Their commitment and enthusiasm emerges through the reading of the chapters.

Patricia Solomon
Sue Baptiste
Hamilton, Ontario
December 2004

Contents

Chapter 3
Strategies for Integrating Basic Sciences in Curriculum

Hallie Groves

Chapter 4
Developing Emerging Roles in Clinical Education

Bonny Jung, Patricia Solomon, Beverley Cole

Chapter 5
Evidence-based Practice for the Rehabilitation Sciences

Patricia Solomon, Lori Letts

Chapter 6
Ethics

E. Lynne Geddes, Margaret Brockett

Chapter 7
Interprofessional Education

Penny Salvatori, Patricia Solomon

Chapter 8
Curricula to Promote Community Health

Julie Richardson, Lori Letts

Chapter 9

Developing Communication Skills

Sue Baptiste, Patricia Solomon

Chapter 10

Developing Community Partnerships

Patricia Solomon, Sue Baptiste

Chapter 11

Evidence-based Admissions in Rehabilitation Science

Penny Salvatori

Chapter 12

Educational Preparation for Rural and Remote Practice: The Northern Studies Stream

Jennifer Cano, Elaine Foster-Seargeant

Chapter 13

A Program Logic Model: A Specific Approach to Curriculum and Program Evaluation

Sue Baptiste, Lori Letts

Directory of Contributors

Sue Baptiste
(e-mail: baptiste@mcmaster.ca)
School of Rehabilitation Science, IAHS – Room 412, McMaster University,
1400 Main St. W., Hamilton, Ontario L8S 1C7, Canada

Margaret Brockett
(e-mail: brocketm@mcmaster.ca)
School of Rehabilitation Science, IAHS – Room 403, McMaster University,
1400 Main St. W., Hamilton, Ontario L8S 1C7, Canada

Jennifer Cano
(e-mail: canoj@mcmaster.ca)
Health Sciences North, Lakehead University, 955 Oliver Road, Thunder Bay,
Ontario, P7B 5E1, Canada

Beverley Cole
(e-mail: colebe@mcmaster.ca)
School of Rehabilitation Science, IAHS – Room 428, McMaster University,
1400 Main St. W., Hamilton, Ontario L8S 1C7, Canada

Elaine Foster-Seargeant
(e-mail: fostere@mcmaster.ca)
Health Sciences North, Lakehead University, 955 Oliver Road, Thunder Bay,
Ontario, P7B 5E1, Canada

E. Lynne Geddes
(e-mail: geddesl@mcmaster.ca)
School of Rehabilitation Science, IAHS – Room 438, McMaster University,
1400 Main St. W., Hamilton, Ontario L8S 1C7, Canada

Hallie Groves
(e-mail: grovesh@mcmaster.ca)
Health Sciences Centre, 1R4, McMaster University, 1200 Main St. W., Hamilton,
Ontario L8N 3Z5, Canada

Bonny Jung
(e-mail: jungb@mcmaster.ca)
School of Rehabilitation Science, IAHS – Room 427, McMaster University,
1400 Main St. W., Hamilton, Ontario L8S 1C7, Canada

Lori Letts
(e-mail: lettsl@mcmaster.ca)
School of Rehabilitation Science, IAHS – Room 436, McMaster University,
1400 Main St. W., Hamilton, Ontario L8S 1C7, Canada

Julie Richardson
(e-mail: jrichard@mcmaster.ca)
School of Rehabilitation Science, IAHS – Room 443, McMaster University,
1400 Main St. W., Hamilton, Ontario L8S 1C7, Canada

Penny Salvatori
(e-mail: salvator@mcmaster.ca)
School of Rehabilitation Science, IAHS – Room 420, McMaster University,
1400 Main St. W., Hamilton, Ontario L8S 1C7, Canada

Patricia Solomon
(e-mail: solomon@mcmaster.ca)
School of Rehabilitation Science, IAHS – Room 437, McMaster University,
1400 Main St. W., Hamilton, Ontario L8S 1C7, Canada

Chapter 1

Skills for the Rehabilitation Professional of the Future

1

Patricia Solomon, Sue Baptiste

Contents

1

Preparing occupational therapy and physiotherapy students for current and future roles in today's complex health care milieu is a formidable challenge for educators. There is an ongoing struggle for educators to find the balance between preparing graduates for the skills for current practice and those required for the future. This battle is in conjunction with ever-increasing demands from professional associations, accreditation and licensing bodies, and the public to add more content to the curriculum.

A focus on content can lead to an overcrowded curriculum and de-emphasize the process of learning. Concerns about an overemphasis on content and of promotion of rote memorization of facts which quickly became outdated, prompted a revolution in medical education. Problem-based learning (PBL), with a focus on the process of learning, started in the medical school at McMaster University in the 1960s. PBL quickly acquired both promoters and critics. In spite of the fact that PBL has been adopted by many medical and health professional schools throughout the world, it continues to receive an unprecedented level of scrutiny and remains controversial. Heated debate abounds within the medical education literature (e.g., Albanese 2000; Colliver 2000; Norman and Schmidt 2000). In this way, PBL has fostered research and debate in medical education and focused attention on educational process and innovation.

While the move to PBL started the debate, educational innovation is not synonymous with PBL. There are now many versions of PBL which have been adapted to fit institutional and professional contexts. There have been calls for curricula and educational methods that promote student-centered learning and the development of life-long learning skills in many professions.

Not surprisingly, this revolution has been somewhat slower to occur within the rehabilitation sciences. During the 1970s and 1980s the occupational therapy and physiotherapy professions were undergoing rapid change with competing priorities for educational innovation. More recently, as roles in the health professions have evolved, there has been a recognized need for curricula which foster the complex skills required for practice in a wide variety of settings (Shepard and Jensen 1990). This book is intended to highlight, support, and illustrate educational innovation. The intent is not solely to promote PBL, but as its philosophical approach emphasizes educational process, there are numerous examples and references to PBL throughout the book. Through sharing our experiences with educational innovation we hope to encourage educators to see the importance of integration of content and process in developing curricula for current and future practice.

New Skills for the Changing Practice Context

The professions of occupational therapy and physiotherapy have evolved at a remarkable pace. Occupational therapy and physiotherapy are relatively young professions that grew out of the needs of the wounded soldiers in the world wars. Roots of the professions are largely traceable to the United Kingdom, although examples of the early manifestations of these disciplines are found within the health care systems in the United States and Canada. Originally, occupational therapy and physiotherapy focused primarily on technical skills, and professional development was under the auspices of the medical profession. As the professions matured, and the need to develop autonomy and a greater scientific foundation for practice became evident, qualifications were advanced to the baccalaureate level. More recently, masters entry level and doctoral entry level degree designations have emerged in response to the need for clinicians who can respond to the increased complexity of current practice environments, the need for advanced skills within an evidenced-based framework, and the need for autonomous practitioners.

Although different countries have varying economic and political pressures, many physiotherapists and occupational therapists today find themselves practicing in an environment with changing demographics, increased accountability, fiscal restraints, increased consumer awareness and expectations, and a shift from institutionally-based to community-based care. Typically, those working within institutional settings no longer have the support provided by a profession-specific departmental structure. This decentralization has meant that therapists have had to increase their non-clinical responsibilities, develop a professional reference group, develop profession-specific quality assurance and risk management, continue external linkages, and develop professional identity and representation (Canadian Physiotherapy Association 2000). The increasing numbers of physiotherapists and occupational therapists working in private practice have had to assume business and marketing responsibilities and develop consultation skills. Fiscal restraints demand that therapists show evidence of cost effectiveness of their treatments. The current push for evidence-based practice requires therapists to keep current with the literature. Hunt et al. (1998) claimed that education should prepare graduates for "professional survival" in the current health care environment. What skills do physiotherapists and occupational therapists need in their "survival kit"?

Self-directed and Lifelong Learning Skills

Recognizing that health professionals work in an environment in which information is rapidly changing, most professional educational programs espouse the importance of developing lifelong learning skills. We agree with Hunt et al. (1998) that developing lifelong learning abilities should be a generic goal of higher education. Candy et al. (quoted in Hunt et al. 1998) have provided a helpful summary of expectations for educational institutions committed to developing lifelong learning skills. These expectations include having an explicit policy on developing lifelong learning, including the development of lifelong learning skills and attitudes as core objectives in all undergraduate courses, and establishing a system for reward and recognition for teaching practices that promote lifelong learning skills.

Although often seen as synonymous with lifelong learning, self-directed learning (SDL) is actually a component of lifelong learning. The development of SDL skills is often a major goal of student-centered innovative curricula. Key elements of SDL require learners to diagnose their learning needs, formulate learning goals, identify appropriate resources for self-study, and evaluate the outcome (Spencer and Jordan 1999).

One of the hallmarks of SDL is the ability to perform accurate self-assessment. The emerging evidence on self-assessment suggests that students are not particularly good at it. For example, Tousignant and DesMarchais (2002) found correlations between third-year medical students' self-assessments of their performance on an oral exam to be low both pre- and post-test. Similarly, Sullivan et al. (1999) found low correlations between faculty and student self-assessment in a PBL course in third-year medical students. Gruppen et al. (2000) note the importance of providing opportunities to develop self-assessment skills. They found that there was no relationship between medical students' self-assessment of their strengths and weaknesses and their allocation of learning time during a third-year clinical clerkship but noted that students had not had time to develop their skills earlier in the curriculum. The studies raise concerns about students' SDL skills: if students cannot self-assess accurately, it seems unlikely that they will be able to determine their gaps in knowledge and skills. Schmidt (2000) also questions the assumption that SDL skills are transferred into professional practice in a commitment to lifelong learning, stating studies pursuing this issue are largely inconclusive. He cautions, however, not to overlook the significant motivational aspects of SDL which are largely related to adult learning theory.

Another skill that is related to SDL is that of critical reflection. The ability to be self-conscious about our actions and to engage in continual self-critique are viewed as critical components of professional competence (Williams 2001). Although the concept of reflection has been in the educational literature for some years, Schön (1987) is widely acknowledged as popularizing the notion in professional practice. The ability to promote reflection in students is enhanced when faculty shift from their role as expert information provider to facilitator of learning. Methods to promote critical reflection are highlighted throughout the book. PBL by its very design fosters reflection. Self-reflective skills are also developed through assignments and evaluations such as reflective journaling, incorporation of self-evaluation and feedback in all educational venues, and critical incident diaries.

Although there are questions related to whether SDL skills developed during professional education transfer into lifelong learning skills after graduation, and whether student-centered curricula promote development of SDL skills better than traditional curricula, we maintain that the overall development of lifelong learning skills should be viewed as an essential component that is incorporated throughout the curriculum. No one would argue that today's health care practitioners must be able to recognize knowledge and skill limitations and have the capacity to determine how to overcome these limitations. It seems reasonable to assume that therapists who engage and practice these skills during their professional education will be better prepared to engage in these practices following graduation. The reinforcement of these skills is implicit in many elements of curriculum design and evaluation throughout this book, and is highlighted in Chapter 2.

Evidence-based Practice Skills

Although the term evidence-based practice (EBP) has become overused and ubiquitous it is an essential element of practice for today's health care practitioners. Current political environments demand that health professionals evaluate the outcomes of their treatments and prove the cost effectiveness of their services. The occupational therapy and physiotherapy professions require ongoing evidence to support their continued growth. In spite of the increasing popularity of EBP, challenges remain in practice as clinicians struggle with trying to incorporate EBP in environments which are "tradition based". Chapter 5 outlines barriers and misconceptions about EBP that are encountered by physiotherapists and occupational therapists and gives examples of how to promote the development of an evidence-based culture throughout a curriculum.

Consultation Skills

As the roles of the physiotherapist and occupational therapist have grown, so has the need to develop consultation skills. While some would argue that consultation skills are beyond entry-level requirements, we believe that several changes in the health care delivery system demand that students are prepared with basic consultation skills upon graduation. A move from departmental structures to program management in institutional settings means that new graduates are often working independently. The health care team does not necessarily view the novice therapist as a "new grad" and depends on his or her expertise to assist in team decision making (Miller et al. 2005). Similarly, the shift from institutionalized care to community-based care and private practice also requires that therapists work independently to develop new roles, educate others, and design and implement programs in response to community need. In addition, the move from medical models to client-centered models of practice focusing on health promotion and disease prevention means that there is a focus on community participation and developing partnerships with clients. It is highly likely that new graduates will encounter the demands resulting from these changes in health care delivery.

There are a number of varying definitions of consultant. We are not suggesting that students are prepared to be "advanced clinical experts", but recognize that they may encounter situations in which they are the sole physiotherapist or occupational therapist and have profession-specific knowledge that needs to be imparted to clients, families, and other members of the health care and social services. Literature in this area is sparse, however there is some evidence that therapists struggle with relinquishing the role of expert and assuming a more consultative role. For example, Litchfield and MacDougall (2002) found that physiotherapists working in the community with children with disabilities and their families were concerned with what they perceived as a loss of "hands on" skills and that the family-centered approach to practice no longer resembled that for which they were trained. Students need to be prepared to assume roles that have their basis in consultation, such as client, family, and community education, working with the community to develop programs which meet its needs, client advocacy, and marketing. Methods to promote these skills are highlighted in the chapters on developing role-emerging clinical placements and on community practice. The challenge for all educators is to ensure that students see these experiences as not only relevant but essential for future practice. It is not uncommon for students to worry about focusing away from hands-on skills as was highlighted in the Litchfield and MacDougall (2002) study.

Communication Skills

Related to consultation skills is the need for educational programs to ensure students develop superior communication skills. A number of trends have necessitated the acquisition of skills beyond those required to develop therapeutic client relationships: the flattening of organizational structures within the institutions has meant that administrative work previously carried out by managers and department heads is often assumed by frontline staff, including new graduates (Miller et al. 2005); supervisory and delegation skills have become essential as cost containment has resulted in greater use of support personnel; the shift to consultative models of care have increased the importance of the therapist's ability to educate and promote health behavior change in clients and their families; and with globalization has come the requirement for health professionals to understand the needs of ethnically diverse groups and adapt their communication style accordingly.

Educational models which encourage students to constructively question each other, debate and justify treatment approaches, and explain and clarify concepts to their colleagues help to promote advanced communication skills. Giving and receiving constructive feedback is a difficult skill that needs to be promoted and role modeled throughout the students' professional education. Chapter 9 discusses how PBL can provide a strong foundation for learning communication skills and presents other alternatives for learning facilitation skills which are helpful in team and client interactions.

It is evident that superior communication skills are required not only for interactions with patients and their families, but also with other members of the health care team. As members of interprofessional teams, both within the community and in institutional settings, therapists must understand the unique contributions and insights of all team members and be able to advocate for their own role. The call for increased emphasis on interprofessional education to promote the understanding of other professional roles and to develop respect and value the input of other health disciplines is not new. In 1988, the World Health Organization (WHO) discussed the importance of interprofessional education and collaborative practice to provide promotive, preventative, curative, rehabilitative, and other health care services. Typically in the debate about essential content in the curriculum, interprofessional learning opportunities, while deemed important, are secondary to other competing areas. Common barriers include inadequate time to plan and implement interprofessional curricula, scheduling difficulties, and faculty attitudes (Larson 1995). There are opposing views on when to introduce interprofessional education (Harden and Davis 1998; van der Horst et al. 1995). Some maintain that interprofessional education should not occur until students have become socialized into their own professional groups suggesting that only senior students should participate. Others suggest that interprofessional education is best targeted to clinical education since that represents the "real" context of professional practice. Chapter 7 explores the literature on interprofessional education and describes some models that have been instituted in the Faculty of Health Sciences at McMaster University.

Professionalism and Ethical Decision Making

With the advent of shifts in the practice environment, there have been increased expectations for professional educational programs to prepare their graduates with a clear appreciation and ownership of the demands of a regulated practice context. Consequently, it is our belief that issues of professionalism and ethical practice should be integrated into the curriculum from the first day to the last. As the disciplines of occupational therapy and physiotherapy emerge into full professions, with the concomitant development of such elements as theoretical practice foundations and adherence to principles of public protection, the demands of practicing in such a complex environment provide a clear imperative to educators to respond. Even during the interview process for program admissions, we draw attention to the need for thinking in a manner conducive to understanding the ethics of being a health professional. As outlined in Chapter 11, during the admissions process applicants are asked to address ethical questions of societal importance, and, once entered into the formal curriculum, this commitment continues. There are many suggested approaches to the "teaching of ethics" and the development of commitment to practicing in an ethical, professional, and conscious manner (Bailey and Schwartzberg 2003; Purtilo 1999). Today's therapists need to develop an innate awareness of their accountability in areas of fiscal management and personal behaviors, and it is the responsibility of the educational process to instill the importance of this foundation of practice within the students and graduates. Chapter 6 describes the ongoing development of ethics content in the occupational therapy and physiotherapy curricula at McMaster University.

Clarity and explication of the expectations of faculty to provide clear role models in these areas are of paramount importance. We believe, therefore, that faculty roles should not be prescribed as having isolated responsibilities for teaching this content, but rather all those providing input into the curriculum should embrace the values of practice in a visible manner, thus providing living lessons for the students to observe, internalize, and emulate. Several chapters within this book address elements of this important area of curricular content.

Barriers to Implementing Innovative Curricula

One of the biggest barriers to implementation of innovative, student-centered curricula are faculty concerns that, when left to their own devices, students will not learn the relevant content. Much of the concern originates in studies which compare medical students' knowledge of the basic sciences across traditional and problem-based curricula. Although findings on comparative studies on tests of knowledge are inconsistent and inconclusive, there is a persistent concern that PBL students will have an insufficient knowledge base, particularly in the basic sciences. While, arguably, the emphasis on basic sciences is somewhat less in the rehabilitation sciences, this sentiment has also been expressed in this literature (Hayes 1998; Jefferson 2001). Several recent studies have had results in favor of PBL. PBL and traditional students from a Canadian medical school performed similarly on their national qualifying exams with the exception of the areas on preventative medicine, psychiatry, and community health where the PBL students scored higher (Kaufman and Mann 1998). Distlehorst and Robbs (1998) found no differences between PBL and traditional medical students on the United States licensing examination. There are few studies in occupational therapy or physiotherapy that shed light on this matter. As this area continues to be controversial we felt it was important to include a chapter which focuses on incorporating basic sciences content in innovative curricula.

In our experience one of the most critical contributors to the success of curriculum renewal is the development of faculty to engage in new roles and invest in the educational endeavor. Many faculty received their professional training in traditional educational settings and have little knowledge in pedagogy or skill in facilitation techniques. Faculty require training to assume more facilitative roles. Hitchcock and Mylona (2000) note that there has been little systematic study on effective ways to train faculty to assume facilitative roles, although there have been many descriptions in the literature. They emphasize that while the most obvious training is in tutor facilitation skills, there are many other roles and skills that need to be developed. Specifically related to PBL, they quote Irby's sequence of steps of skill development: (1) challenging

1

assumptions and developing understanding of PBL, (2) experiencing and valuing the tutorial process, (3) acquiring general tutor skills, (4) developing content-specific tutor knowledge and skills, (5) acquiring advanced knowledge and skills, (6) developing leadership and scholarship skills, and (7) creating organizational vitality.

Within the medical education literature there has been considerable study of whether content experts or educational process experts are preferable in small group problem-based tutorial settings. Dolmans et al. (2001) provided an excellent summary of issues related to tutor expertise in a recent review. Not surprisingly, a combination of both content and process experts was determined to be preferable.

The skills required by the tutor may vary according to the level of the students. Qualitative studies in both occupational therapy (Hammel et al. 1999) and physiotherapy (Solomon and Finch 1998) found that students experienced considerable anxiety in adapting to more student-centered curricula. Students lacked confidence in their ability to adapt, misunderstood the faculty role, worried about learning cooperatively in a group setting, and about conducting self-evaluation and providing feedback to other group members. This suggests that tutors who are facilitating PBL neophytes need group process and facilitation skills to assist in the initial adjustment phase.

The costs associated with the faculty time required to deliver education in small groups is another key concern and potential barrier to implementation (Albanese and Mitchell 1993). Other costs relate to space requirements for small group tutorial rooms and development of self-directed learning resources (Solomon et al. 1992). Without institutional support for curricular change, many programs may find it difficult to engage successfully in curriculum reform.

One final barrier to the implementation of innovative curricula relates to the lack of rigorous long-term data which demonstrate significant differences between more traditional and innovative curricula. Most outcome studies have compared medical students in PBL and non-PBL curricula. If we are to learn from our medical colleagues it may not be practical or affordable to implement studies which evaluate different curricular models. Comparative studies are complex, multifactorial, and fraught with methodological challenges making it difficult to attribute differences solely to the curriculum. However, reflecting and reporting on our experiences is an essential building block for ongoing curricular innovation to address the ever-changing needs for educational preparation of occupational therapists and physiotherapists.

Conclusion

The changing practice environment with the resultant increase in expectations for entry-level occupational therapists and physiotherapists challenges educators to produce skilled clinicians who can react to change, integrate evidence into clinical decision making, communicate effectively, educate and consult to their clients and the health care team, and assume administrative responsibilities. These skills cannot be developed solely through traditional faculty-centered teaching methods and demand that educators examine their process through which education occurs. Through this book we share experiences and examples of educational innovation that have been the cornerstone of the occupational therapy and physiotherapy curricula at McMaster University.

References

Albanese M (2000) Problem-based learning: why curricula are likely to show little effect on knowledge and clinical skills. Med Educ 34:729–738

Albanese MA, Mitchell S (1993) Problem-based learning: a review of literature on its outcomes and implementation issues. Acad Med 68:52–81

Bailey DM, Schwartzberg SL (2003) Ethical and legal dilemmas in occupational therapy. Davis, Philadelphia

Canadian Physiotherapy Association (2000) Health care restructuring: a resource manual for physiotherapists. Canadian Physiotherapy Association, Toronto

Colliver JA (2000) Effectiveness of problem-based learning: research and theory. Acad Med 75:259–266

Distlehorst LH, Robbs RS (1998) A comparison of problem-based learning and standard curriculum students: three years of retrospective data. Teach Learn Med 10:131–137

Dolmans DHJM, Wolfhagen IHAP, Scherpbier AJJA, van der Vleuten CPM (2001) Relationship of tutors' group-dynamics skills to their performance ratings in problem-based learning. Acad Med 76:473–476

Gruppen LD, White C, Fitzgerald JT, Grum CM, Woolliscroft JO (2000) Medical students' self-assessments and their allocations of learning time. Acad Med 75:374–379

Hammel J, Royeen CB, Bagatell N, Chandler B, Jensen G, Loveland J, Stone G (1999) Student perspectives on problem-based learning in an occupational therapy curriculum: a multiyear qualitative study. Am J Occup Ther 53:199–206

Harden RM, Davis MH (1998) The continuum of problem-based learning. Med Teach 20:317–322

Hayes SH (1998) Invited commentary. Phys Ther 78:207–209

Hitchcock MA, Mylona Z (2000) Teaching faculty to conduct problem-based learning. Teach Learn Med 12:52–57

Hunt A, Adamson B, Higgs J, Harris L (1998) University education and the physiotherapy professional. Physiotherapy 84:264–273

Jefferson JR (2001) Problem-based learning and the promotion of problem solving: choices for physical therapy curricula. J Phys Ther Educ 15:26–31

Kaufman DM, Mann KV (1998) Comparing achievement on the Medical Council of Canada Qualifying Examination Part I of students in conventional and problem-based learning curricula. Acad Med 73:1211–1213

Larson E (1995) New rules for the game: interdisciplinary education for health professionals. Nurs Outlook 43:180–185

Litchfield R, MacDougall C (2002) Professional issues for physiotherapists in family centred and community based settings. Aust J Physiother 48:105–112

Miller P, Solomon P, Giacomini M, Abelson J (2005) Experiences of novice physiotherapists adapting to their role in acute care hospitals. Physiother Can 57:1–9

Norman GR, Schmidt HG (2000) Effectiveness of problem-based learning: theory, practice and paper darts. Med Educ 34:721–728

Purtilo R (1999) Ethical dimensions in the health professions. Saunders, Philadelphia

Schmidt H (2000) Assumptions underlying self-directed learning may be false. Med Educ 34:243–245

Schön D (1987) Educating the reflective practitioner: toward a new design for teaching and learning in the professions. Jossey-Bass, San Francisco

Shepard K, Jensen G (1990) Physical therapy curricula for the 1990s: educating the reflective practitioner. Phys Ther 70:566–577

Solomon P, Finch E (1998) A qualitative study identifying stressors associated with adapting to problem-based learning. Teach Learn Med 10:58–64

Solomon P, Blumberg P, Shehata A (1992) The influence of patient age on problem-based learning discussion. Acad Med 67:531–533

Spencer JA, Jordan RK (1999) Learner centred approaches in medical education. BMJ 318:1280–1283

Sullivan ME, Hitchcock MA, Dunnington GL (1999) Peer and self assessment during problem-based tutorial. Am J Surg 177:266–269

1

Tousignant M, DesMarchais JE (2002) Accuracy of student self-assessment ability compared to their own performance in a problem-based learning medical program: a correlation study. Adv Health Sci Educ 7:19–27

Van der Horst M, Turpie I, Nelson W, Cole B, Sammon S, Sniderman P, Tremblay M (1995) St. Joseph's Community Health Center model of community-based interdisciplinary health care team education. Health Soc Care Community 3:33–42

Williams B (2001) Developing critical reflection for professional practice through problem-based learning. J Adv Nurs 34:27–34

World Health Organization (1988) Learning together to work together for health. WHO, Geneva (Technical report series, vol 769

Chapter 2

Curriculum Development and Design

2

Sue Baptiste, Patricia Solomon

2

A historical overview of the physiotherapy and occupational therapy programs at McMaster University will assist in providing a context for the discussions within this chapter. During the late 1960s and early 1970s, programs in both physiotherapy and occupational therapy were established at Mohawk College in Hamilton, Ontario. These programs arose from the thinking of a group of pioneers who believed that the educational approach that had been developed by medical education innovators at McMaster University was also most relevant for the preparation of occupational therapists and physiotherapists. Consequently, a group of educators from both institutions, Mohawk College and McMaster University, combined their skills and created a vision that became the diploma programs in occupational therapy and physiotherapy. This approach was problem-based learning, and was used as the foundation for both programs from their inception to the present day, across three different iterations of curriculum. One of the key innovations to the way in which the college programs were taught was the combination of using faculty from both the university and college to teach all courses. In the 1980s, a degree completion program was launched that provided graduates of the diploma program a chance to upgrade their qualification to a bachelors degree from McMaster University. This was particularly important since the minimum credential for entry to practice had been raised to the baccalaureate level by the professional associations. In 1989, the program moved completely into the university setting and the graduates were granted a BHSc(PT) or BHSc(OT), a bachelor degree in health sciences. Ten years later, in 2000, candidates were admitted to the entry-level masters programs in occupational therapy and physiotherapy.

The Pedagogical Framework: Problem-based Learning

As briefly referred to above, the occupational therapy and physiotherapy programs at McMaster University have a strong history with and legacy of problem-based learning. While the initial curriculum models were strongly influenced by the inaugural undergraduate medical curriculum, time and confidence presented opportunities to create our own models. These models reflect the special nuances of each discipline.

Problem-based learning is recognized as having begun at McMaster University, in the medical curriculum, and was in response to critical concerns about the nature of more traditional learning models in medical curricula. The intention was to create an approach to teaching and learning that was learner-centered, yet based upon clear objectives and evaluation criteria. The key difference was the expectation that learners would be facilitated and guided rather than taught (Barrows and Tamblyn 1980; Neufeld 1983; Saarinen and Salvatori 1994). Both the occupational therapy and physiotherapy programs at McMaster University have embraced these ideas, although with differing degrees of connection and commitment to the original model. In fact, true problem-based learning models should naturally emerge from each individual context and culture. There is no "right" way although there is a growing recognition of a common set of principles and elements that can be applied to determine the "problem-based-ness" of a learning environment (Maudesley 1994; Walton and Matthews 1989). Problem-based learning principles tend to become grouped in two distinct categories: first, the values upon which problem-based learning is based and second, some characteristics that are held in common understanding as being critical to the core of problem-based learning. Underlying values include: partnership, honesty and openness, mutual respect, and trust. Core characteristics incorporate:

- Learning which is student/learner-centered
- Faculty roles that are those of facilitator and guide
- Learning scenarios which form the basis, focus, and stimulus for learning
- New information and understanding that is acquired through self-directed learning (Baptiste 2003 p. 17)

Consequently, there is a continuum of problem-based curricula from pure through hybrid models. The masters entry-level physiotherapy and occupational therapy programs at the School of Rehabilitation Science at McMaster University continue to be based upon problem-based principles. Although both programs are very different one from the other, there are also many common elements and approaches that are celebrated. Examples of these similarities are cited throughout this book, particularly in the chapters focusing on evidence-based practice and ethics education.

Approaching the Task of Curriculum Renewal

Perhaps one of the most overwhelming, yet exciting, tasks with which to be confronted is the opportunity and challenge of developing a new curriculum. This task is made even more daunting when circumstances provide a chance to do something different based on external forces and not a need to change because "something is broken". Over the past few years, and in several years to come, many educational programs in rehabilitation science are facing this situation. The changing nature of the entry-level credential for occupational therapists and physiotherapists demands that faculty undertake a detailed review of curricula, to determine the optimal approach to moving toward graduate-level preparation, or, at the very least, complete a review of existing curricula models to identify their responsiveness and congruence with emerging practice expectations and demands.

Approaches to such a massive task can vary from ensuring the preservation of what is good from the existing curriculum to making a total shift and adopting a radically

Table 2.1. Principles for curricular change and innovation

Rationale should be articulated explicitly
Overall goals should be reiterated constantly throughout the process
Continuing communication is essential, coupled with a clear rationale
Ensure that the intended change is in response to a defined and recognized need or purpose
Ensure that the innovation is seen as a high institutional priority
Focus on pedagogy and not on resources for implementation
Foster strong leadership support
Identify incentives for faculty participation
Gain faculty buy-in for the curricular blueprint
Involve the active teaching faculty throughout the process
Anticipate potential barriers to change and develop strategies to address them
Recognize the potential need for and value of negotiation

Adapted from Guze (1995)

2

new approach and design. To have an optimal effect, options to be considered should bear relevance to the pervading culture of the institution and environment within which the curriculum is to thrive. Also, decisions must be made concerning the pedagogical choices of how learner-centered the curriculum should be, and what particular educational modalities are the best for the circumstances.

This chapter will address the entire picture of curriculum development and design, from the first conversations about how to engage in the renewal process through making decisions about methods of teaching, approaches to learner assessment, and preparation of entry-level practitioners for the emerging practice contexts.

Guze (1995) provided a clear and succinct discussion of several core principles that can guide curricular change and innovation (Table 2.1). The following is an overview of these principles.

Where to Begin?

Motivation for curriculum renewal can come from both internal and external forces. External expectations from regulatory and professional bodies are tending to impose standards for new practitioners that require:

- Preparation at an advanced level of clinical reasoning and judgment
- The ability to assume roles that require autonomy and a strong sense of professional ethics
- Engaging in their professional role from the first day of practice, in a conscious and moral manner that requires reflection and self-awareness

Regardless of whether the motivation for curricular change stems from a desire to do something differently or better, or from outside influences, the task is one that requires careful planning. However, it is imperative that any planning process recognizes the need to dream and envision what could be, to create a model that will exemplify those visions, and to produce a graduate who is well prepared to face the complexities and challenges of emerging practice.

When developing a curriculum, four general questions must be asked:

- What is the purpose of the curriculum?
- What educational experiences can be created to fulfill this purpose?
- What is the most effective manner in which to organize these educational experiences?
- How can we determine that the purpose has been fulfilled and the goals attained (Wiers et al. 2002)?

Another very critical element of any change is the recognition that the cultural context is a key in managing change successfully. Hafferty (1998), when reflecting upon the realities of a medical school curriculum, discusses the existence of informal and hidden curricula as well as the formal curriculum. He posits that, in order to induce a lasting change, the entire organizational culture needs to be engaged to facilitate students and faculty alike in embracing and working with change. When facing the task of curricular reform, redesign has to occur not only in terms of content, but also in relation to the educational processes that enable the learning to take place. This is the difference between reforming the syllabus and reforming the curriculum; the overall learning environment of the educational program and institution is changed (Burton and McDonald 2001).

Once the decision has been made to reform the curriculum, a first step is to complete an environmental scan and situational analysis that explore the educational and organizational environment within the institution, to determine what will facilitate the proposed changes. By defining a clear and newly articulated set of priorities and guidelines, changes that are being made within the curriculum will be given the vehicle through which impact can be made upon the surrounding environment (Genn 2001). This strategy is part of the first overall phase, *the planning phase*. This is when the need for change is established and the vision for change is designed. It is during this phase of development that the non-negotiable elements of structure and process are determined. For example, within the School of Rehabilitation Science at McMaster University, both the Physiotherapy and Occupational Therapy Programs were already designed as two-year, twenty-four-month, curricula. Also, the province of Ontario mandates that all masters programs are two years in duration. Therefore, the decision was readily made, based on these graduate program regulations and history, that the new masters entry-level curricula would be twenty-four months long. One key commitment was clear and that was to the foundational philosophy of problem-based, self-directed learning utilizing the application of these principles to small group, large group, and skills-based learning experiences.

Wiers et al. (2002) provide a clear and helpful outline of ten general steps of curriculum design within a problem-based learning context (see Table 2.2). While this rubric is structured around the specific processes inherent within problem-based learning development, most of the guidelines can apply broadly across any curricular development process within any pedagogical framework.

From the onset, all faculty members at McMaster University were on board regarding the need to undertake the development of entry-level masters curricula in both occupational therapy and physiotherapy. Both disciplines had undergone dramatic changes in the preceding two decades, largely focused upon the growth of foundational science and evidence for practice. Professional practice models had emerged for both professions and provided a strong backdrop against which to create fresh ap-

Table 2.2. Ten general steps in curriculum design for a problem-based learning (PBL) environment

1. Give rationale for the curriculum and form a planning group
2. Generate general educational objectives for the curriculum
3. Assess the educational needs of future students
4. Apply general principles of PBL to the curriculum
5. Structure the curriculum and generate a curriculum blueprint
6. Elaborate the unit blueprints
7. Construct the study units
8. Decide on student assessment methods
9. Consider the educational organization and curriculum management model
10. Evaluate the curriculum and revise as appropriate

Adapted from Wiers et al. (2002)

proaches to the preparation of graduates for entering practice. While both the occupational therapy and physiotherapy programs undertook curriculum renewal at the same time, the physiotherapy program had engaged in an ongoing process of change across the preceding five years. Many of the issues, concerns, and changes addressed and implemented by the occupational therapy program had already been addressed by physiotherapy. Therefore, this chapter will focus predominantly upon the initiatives inherent within the curricular shift within occupational therapy, although reference will be made to processes within physiotherapy as appropriate.

Designing Our New Programs

Deciding upon the overarching constructs that would determine the final curriculum model was a complex and dramatic process in many ways, and one in which everyone was eager to participate and have a chance to have input.

At the onset of the development of the occupational therapy program, three faculty retreats were held that progressed from a totally unstructured brainstorm of what would be perfect, to a detailed accounting of core curricular elements in the context of a delivery structure. In the initial retreat, all full-time faculty members together with some part-time members participated in a "blue-skying" day-long session during which everyone spoke of their dreams for the perfect curriculum. What if we could do what we wanted? What if we did not have to be concerned with logistics like room bookings? – and so on. This exercise provided us with a high-level appreciation of the values and elements that were important to us as a collective. It was from this beginning "fantasy" that the next level of planning emerged. The second retreat was more structured and focused upon the creation of a continuum for learning that resulted in the overarching framework for the curriculum, together with the delivery methods. A process was followed whereby we decided upon a central construct around which the whole curriculum would evolve, namely, "occupation". To support this core notion, there were several longitudinal conceptual threads that represented continua of thought such as: wellness to illness, simplicity to complexity, local to global, and unifaceted to multifaceted. Through this process, we were able to identify the starting place for the first study term, and to create a high-level framework for the progression of the total curriculum (see Table 2.3)

In physiotherapy, the process began similarly with a faculty retreat; however, the focus varied slightly. Initial discussions identified elements of the curriculum that we

Table 2.3. Occupational therapy curricular framework

Term	Content theme
1	Wellness, health, and occupation
2	Person, environment, and occupation
3	Development, disability, and occupation
4	Youth and the development of self
5	Adulthood and disability
6	Complexities of contemporary practice

valued and wanted to maintain and those needing less emphasis. Through ongoing curricular evaluation and feedback, we identified new areas that needed to be included in the emerging curriculum and other areas that needed to be enhanced. These areas were discussed within the context of the changing practice of physiotherapy and the knowledge and skills required by the physiotherapist in the new millennium. The decision was made to use a curricular framework that incorporated a modified "body systems" design, as current physiotherapy practice and clinical specialties were aligned with this model. Inclusion of a Community Practice/Community Health unit allowed for a focus on emergent health care roles in the community and on integrating health promotion and disease prevention into practice. The faculty recognized that while many physiotherapists identified their practice in an area related to the body systems, increasingly clinicians were faced with more complex patients with multiple system involvement. Hence, the final unit of study focused on integrated practice dealing with clients with complex multisystem health care problems.

Following the initial planning process, it is now time to initiate the plan. It is during this time period that the "unfreezing" of old organizational patterns and the introduction of innovations into the educational environment take place (Burton and McDonald 2001). Often, while there is a strong commitment to engaging in the conversations that lead to the design of a changed reality, it is a very different matter to start "doing" and actually making that changed reality come to life. A cooperative internal environment is essential for the realization of that initial dream and therefore it is well worthwhile for planners to engage in a transparent and collaborative experience that enables maximum participation and open debate. A process of this nature is characterized by collaborative problem solving, effective communication, abilities in conflict resolution, and a cultural expectation of working together in harmony that guides the overall enterprise (Burton and McDonald 2001). Therefore, it is of importance to determine at the onset the values and behaviors by which the development experience will be approached to set up structures and processes that will ensure that the best attempts at making it so will be expended.

During the initiation period, we experienced intense interest and levels of emotion from all participants regarding the manner in which the planning and the visions for the two disciplines would be evolved and realized. As mentioned previously, we had determined that the existing problem-based learning principles would remain but that the key changes would be realized through the manner in which the content was introduced to the students and through which the continuum of learning would evolve. Similarly, we were committed to maintaining a student-centered approach. One core difference was to be the manner in which the experiential component of professional preparation would be integrated more centrally into both curricula. Previously, the curricula were designed in a more traditional fashion whereby the clinical fieldwork experiences were placed at the end of each study term and were linked directly to the area of academic focus for the preceding learning block. By definition, once the overarching concepts of the curricula were determined to be different from the previous models, then fieldwork placements would become less strictly aligned. This was reinforced more heavily in the occupational therapy program which was originally designed around developmental stages and central practice populations. Students would face a more eclectic approach in their clinical learning; therefore, both programs determined that learning around professional issues and practice expectations should be interwoven through the longitudinal axis of the curriculum.

2

Redevelopment Within a Problem-based Learning Culture

As with any problem-based learning system, the small group learning unit is the nucleus of the whole curriculum. However, the success of problem-based, small group learning is supported by the strategic use of large group interactions for the imparting of theoretical and expert knowledge, while still maintaining a problem-based learning philosophy. Similarly, the application of problem-based learning principles is a critical piece of one-on-one learning and synthesis of knowledge and information throughout the academic and clinical components of the curriculum overall. Both the physiotherapy and occupational therapy programs elected to continue to utilize problem-based learning methods in a manner that celebrated the development already achieved over twenty-five years of curriculum development. This has evolved over time very differently in each program. For example, during the planning process for the occupational therapy curriculum, efforts were made to define new models for tutoring and many were identified and put into place. During the second year of the occupational therapy program, the problem-based tutorials occur only once weekly. This allows additional scheduling time for including the evidence-based practice courses and is also in response to the difficulties many practitioners are experiencing in gaining release time from employers to participate as tutors. In this new tutorial model, tutors are required to participate in only one weekly session with two or three tutors' meetings across the term instead of weekly.

Application of problem-based learning principles in large groups has been maintained and, in fact, enhanced particularly in the clinical skills sessions. Students often are placed in small groups (different groups from their core tutorial group) and provided with opportunities to explore assessment tools and intervention methods. Through these group experiences, the students apply a problem-based learning approach to the identification of learning issues, the uncovering of essential information and resources, and the synthesis of their understanding of the tool or technique.

Integration of Experiential Practice Preparation Within a Problem-based Learning Framework

As mentioned earlier, both the physiotherapy and occupational therapy faculty groups were committed to ensuring the integration of academic and experiential learning into the curricula from the beginning, and were focused on developing innovative models for the synthesis of practice preparation into the core academic units. It is important to note that the work related to integration commenced at the very onset of the curriculum planning process. In the case of the occupational therapy program, there had always been sessions held throughout the full curriculum that provided opportunities for the Clinical Placement Coordinator (now Professional Practice Coordinator) to inform, advise, educate, and monitor students in preparing for their practice experiences and in checking in with them following these experiences. However, a greater focus on such integration was placed within the masters entry-level curriculum model in order to ensure that students were being prepared to meet the enhanced expectations of a graduate program.

Evaluation Within a Graduate Problem-based Learning Framework

There should be clear and close linkages between how students learn and how that learning is assessed. Therefore, some information will be presented here relative to the evaluation methods developed at McMaster University in the occupational therapy and physiotherapy programs.

■ **Student Evaluation.** In the preceding years, the two programs at McMaster University had been very involved in designing evaluation/student assessment tools that reflected the principles of problem-based learning and provided students with opportunities to integrate their academic learning with their growing professional awareness and identity. Most of these tools are built around the basic problem-based learning process of exploring a learning scenario that has been developed to address the objectives for the particular learning unit. Essentially, problem-based evaluation needs to be congruent with the underlying values and principles of problem-based learning. Traditional methods of assessing students' knowledge tend to be contradictory to these principles and therefore should not be applied out of context. Problem-based learner assessment should:

- Be congruent with the underlying problem-based learning process illustrated by the development of learning scenarios based on real life practice situations

- Mirror the problem-based learning process of reflecting on a practice scenario, defining learning issues, researching, synthesizing, and synopsizing the learning with application to the defined case

- Involve personal reflection and enhanced awareness of individual critical thinking and clinical reasoning skills

■ **Faculty Evaluation.** As with student assessment, the evaluation of faculty is central to the maintenance and enhancement of a problem-based learning culture. And, similarly, faculty evaluation is built into the roles played in any given learning context. In the case of the small group tutor role, faculty members are evaluated by each student and provide a self-evaluation to students during the course of the group process. Following the completion of the small group experience, students evaluate the faculty member as well as the overall course, and these ratings are provided to faculty and placed in their file for attention at times when promotion, tenure, and merit increase decisions are made. For those faculty members, practitioners, and others who facilitate large group sessions in both theory and practical skills, similar evaluations are completed. This process has been in place over many years and has not changed since the advent of the new curricula. However, the items being evaluated have altered to reflect the expected level and scope of graduate teaching.

■ **Student Self-assessment: Development of the OTPPI.** Students admitted into the occupational therapy program are not expected to have any prerequisite courses completed during their undergraduate education. This has been the case from the very beginning. In the program itself, there are no formal courses that provide students with basic knowledge related to the foundational sciences that underlie occupational therapy practice such as anatomy, physics, biochemistry, sociology, psychology, and anthropology. It has been the long-held belief that in a pure problem-based learning environment, the learning is accomplished through the horizontal meshing of various areas of knowledge and information; that through the integration of these sciences and bodies of knowledge, students can gain the understanding they require by using real life situations as springboards for integration and synthesis of all inputs. Consequently, recent efforts were expended to develop the Occupational Therapy Personal Progress Inventory (OTPPI), a tool that was developed from the experience of the undergraduate medical program over the past few years (Blake et al. 1996; Cunnington 2001). The OTPPI focuses on foundational knowledge that our students need in order to become practicing occupational therapists. It is not a test of the application of that knowledge in practice. The examination consists of 90 multiple-choice questions developed with the expectation that a "star" student would be able to answer by the time of graduation. There are three main domains included in each examination: biology (this includes anatomy, physiology, etc.), social sciences (this includes psychology, sociology, anthropology, etc.), and research (this includes statistics, research methods, ethics, etc.). The breakdown of each examination is 40 percent biology, 40 percent social science, and 20 percent research. The examination is generated each term and students in both years have the same examination, with the expectation that the students in second year will achieve a higher result than those in the first year. Students receive a detailed report with their scores and a profile of how they have progressed over time. They are provided with information about their total score as well as a breakdown on each of the three domains. They also receive a zone score, which is an indication of how well they have performed on the test in comparison to the other members of the class. Students in the yellow or red zones may want to review their scores in more detail and make learning plans to address gaps that may have been identified through the examination. This tool is designed as a self-assessment measure, the individual results of which are known only to each student. We have made a conscious choice that results are not used in the summative evaluation of the students, and are intended to provide the learners with a sense of how they are progressing in accumulating knowledge relative to the basic sciences of their discipline. The students are expected to use that information to set plans in place to address weaknesses (e.g., through problem-based tutorials, individual assignments, etc.). The OTPPI has been a pencil and paper test so far, but steps are being taken to convert it to a web-based format. While the occupational therapy program has undertaken this initiative on a pilot basis, initial responses would indicate that students are finding the process helpful to them, although this is very new at the time of publication.

■ **Integration of Evidence-based Practice Skills into the Curricula.** The integration of skills related to practicing in an evidence-based manner is seen to be critical to both programs. A detailed description of the models adopted by the occupational therapy and physiotherapy programs is found in Chapter 5. In both programs, there is a strong commitment to evidence-based practice as a central construct for the curriculum and a natural partner for client-centered and problem-based principles.

Conclusion

Since their inception, the masters entry-level programs in occupational therapy and physiotherapy have presented opportunities to revisit our history and legacy in health sciences education. In order to reflect on the overall process, the general steps for curriculum design offered by Wiers et al. (2002) will be revisited (see Table 2.2).

For us, the *rationale for the curriculum* was clear both from an internal and an external perspective, and the notion of *forming a planning group* was a natural approach to the task. Our profound commitment to involving our broad academic community was illustrated through the involvement of a wide range of individuals encompassing full-time, part-time, and sessional faculty members as well as members of the wider practice community. Such involvement was realized throughout the planning process and continues through such individuals' representation on our Education, Curriculum and Admissions committees. The need to define clear *general educational objectives for the curriculum* was also recognized at a very early stage. We found that being able to determine the goals and directions from the outset served to facilitate the planning that followed. *Assessing the educational needs of future students* was assisted by our own knowledge concerning the entry-level competencies demanded by our professional regulatory colleges. Also, the connections we have with our practice communities and past graduates were invaluable in providing a background for determining the shifts necessary within the curriculum to fulfill practice expectations. Similarly, the same thoughtful reasoning was used to consider the differences of teaching and learning between undergraduate and graduate approaches to education.

Applying general principles of problem-based learning to the curriculum was not a concern for us, given our long history of internalizing this philosophy. Specific difficulties arose when converting the undergraduate courses and assessment tools to the needs of a graduate program. Nevertheless, problem-based learning in many ways is a gift for this transition since it resembles closely the natural proclivities of graduate work – smaller groups, self-directedness, learner autonomy, and a degree of freedom to determine learning directions.

Structuring the curriculum and creating a blueprint became different experiences for physiotherapy and occupational therapy. As mentioned previously, while the planning processes looked ostensibly similar, the manner in which the final curricular models were derived was very different (see Tables 2.3 and 2.4). However, after the master models were created, the processes for *elaborating the blueprints* and *constructing study units* were again very similar. Methods of *student assessment* tended to remain grounded in the familiar processes and tools that we had developed across our history with problem-based learning. However, as each curricular element emerged throughout the planning (e.g., evidence-based practice, ethics, clinical skills, fieldwork) so did innovative ways to enhance the student assessment processes that were already strong. Details of these innovations will be discussed in the book chapters relating to these specific areas.

Consideration of the educational organization and curriculum management model required particular attention since our lines of accountability had shifted, with the

Table 2.4. Physiotherapy curricular framework

Unit	Content theme
1	Fundamentals of physiotherapy practice
2	Fundamentals of musculoskeletal practice
3	Fundamentals of cardiorespiratory and neurological practice
4	Advanced neurological practice
5	Community practice
6	Integrated practice and professional transition

2

move to the School of Graduate Studies. Two slightly different models of governance emerged, with the Admissions Committee being the only shared group between physiotherapy and occupational therapy. However, both governance models reflect a central group responsible and accountable for curriculum and another group that oversees general program functioning.

Curricular evaluation remains an ongoing responsibility and expectation. Chapter 13 provides a particular model for curriculum evaluation that was used by the occupational therapy program, the Program Logic Model. However, there are many ways in which faculty members can retain a clear image of what makes up a curriculum and what indicators are critical to evaluate for the success of the program overall.

The three years of planning and launching the new curricula at McMaster University were years of extremely hard work, high energy and output. As we see each student cohort graduate, and receive feedback concerning our students and graduates in practice settings, we feel heartened that we appear to be on the right track. We know, however, that curriculum development is an ongoing process. We also know that curriculum design must be fluid and flexible enough to withstand challenges and changes that come from internal and external sources.

References

Baptiste S (2003) Problem-based learning: a self-directed journey. Slack, Thorofare, NJ

Barrows HS, Tamblyn RM (1980) Problem-based learning: an approach to medical education. Springer, Berlin Heidelberg New York (Medical education, vol 1)

Blake JM, Norman GR, Keane DR, Mueller CB, Cunnington JPW, Didyk N (1996) Introducing progress testing in McMaster University's problem-based medical curriculum: psychometric properties and effect on learning. Acad Med 71:1002–1007

Burton JL, McDonald S (2001) Curriculum or syllabus: which are we reforming? Med Teach 23: 187–191

Cunnington J (2001) Evolution of student evaluation in the McMaster MD programme. Pedagogue 10, Program for Educational Research and Development, Faculty of Health Sciences, McMaster University, Hamilton, ON

Genn JM (2001) AMEE Medical Education Guide no. 23 (part 1): curriculum, environment, climate, quality and change in medical education – a unifying perspective. Med Teach 23: 337–344

Guze PA (1995) Cultivating curricular reform. Acad Med 70:971–973

Hafferty FW (1998) Beyond curriculum reform: confronting medicine's hidden curriculum. Acad Med 73:403–407

Maudesley G (1994) Do we all mean the same thing by "problem-based learning"?: a review of the concepts and a formulation of the ground rules. Acad Med 74:178–185

Neufeld VR (1983) Adventures of an adolescent: curriculum changes at McMaster University. In: Friedman C, Purcell ES (eds) New biology and medical education. Josiah Macy Jr Foundation, New York, pp 256–270

Saarinen H, Salvatori P (1994) Dialogue: educating occupational and physiotherapists for the year 2000: what, no anatomy courses? Physiother Can 46:81–86

Walton HJ, Matthews MB (1989) Essentials of problem-based learning. Med Educ 23:542–558

Wiers RW, van de Wiel MWJ, Sa HLC, Mamede S, Tomaz JB, Schmidt HG (2002) Design of a problem-based curriculum: a general approach and a case study in the domain of public health. Med Teach 24:45–51

Chapter 3

Strategies for Integrating Basic Sciences in Curriculum

3

Hallie Groves

Contents

3

Educational programs aimed at preparing health care practitioners for professional practice present particular challenges when attempting to optimize the learning of basic sciences content. The core issue is the need to focus this learning at a level that is relevant to the knowledge required for the profession in question. Ideally the basic sciences content in a health professional curriculum should enable students to achieve an appropriate level of knowledge and understanding, and to appreciate the relevance and application of their learning to their future practice.

In conventional curricula, basic sciences such as anatomy and physiology are usually presented in a traditional lecture and laboratory format. Not uncommonly, students focus their learning on what is needed to pass the course, while giving little thought to the relevance or application of the information to their professional practice. A traditional anatomy course often includes a "tour of duty" for students during which time is spent in many rigorous hours of dissection, lectures, and immersion in texts memorizing names of structures, origins and insertions of muscles, and so on.

In a clinical program, students' knowledge and understanding of the basic sciences should become a dynamic, integral part of their thinking, reasoning, and problem solving. Ultimately the student should become a lifelong learner able to appreciate the importance of advancements in the basic sciences and how they apply to clinical practice . Integrating the basic sciences into an innovative, student-centered curriculum can be an effective strategy for facilitating learning and ensuring that the students appreciate the clinical relevance of the material. A well-designed problem or scenario can provide a powerful stimulus for learning. Because the learning is occurring in the context of the problem, there is an increased emphasis on learning and applying the new knowledge. This not only increases the focus on the most important content, but also facilitates the attainment of an appropriate depth and breadth of knowledge and understanding. There is good evidence that problem-based learning (PBL) results in a level of basic sciences knowledge no different from that of students in traditional programs (Prince et al. 2003). In addition, students using PBL achieve a deeper understanding of important information (Coles 1985; Newble and Clarke 1986).

The issues that must be addressed to provide an active learning experience in basic sciences include:

- what to learn and how to organize it
- The selection of appropriate learning resources
- The role of the faculty
- The ability to facilitate active learning in the students
- The appropriate evaluation of the knowledge

Basic Sciences in an Integrated Curriculum: What to Learn?

One of the most difficult challenges in determining the basic sciences content for a curriculum is to decide what the students really "need to know and understand." Do the students need a very broad base of knowledge to form a foundation for future learning, an in-depth knowledge and understanding in a focused area, or both? What facts, concepts, processes, level of knowledge, and understanding of application are required? Ensuring that the active learner covers the desired curriculum is a challenge (MacLeod 1999; Sweeney 1999).

may be designed to integrate or link information from several different subject areas. Modules are linked together to support learning of related information.

Example: A group of modules on the musculoskeletal system could be designed to integrate information on skeletal development, congenital anomalies, gross anatomy, histology, physiology, radiology, and assessment of patients. One of the modules could include specimens of bone or joint pathology, X-rays of diseased joints, resources related to assessment and treatment, and references to recent publications and research. Another module could be designed to help a student develop an understanding of the brachial plexus and innervation of the upper limb. A section on brachial plexus and upper limb nerve injuries could include common sites of injury, the possible mechanisms responsible and the effects of particular injuries on motor function, as well as assessment, treatment, and prognosis. This could be presented as a series of clinical cases such as a baby that suffered a brachial plexus injury during birth, a man who was involved in an industrial accident that resulted in a severe injury to his ulnar nerve at the elbow, or a computer programmer who developed carpal tunnel syndrome.

There are a large number of professionally *dissected specimens* or "prosections" in the anatomy laboratory at McMaster University. The collection includes, for example, a range of both superficial and deeper dissections of large specimens of the thorax, abdomen, limbs, back, head and neck, as well as smaller specimens of organs and joints. The specimens are indexed and available in the laboratory throughout the year so that students or faculty can quickly access the anatomical structures or region of interest.

Example: There are over 15 prosections of the knee. The superficial dissections show structures such as veins and cutaneous nerves, while the deeper dissections show muscle layers, tendons, arteries, joint capsule, ligaments, bursae, menisci, and articular surfaces. These specimens can be accessed by individuals or groups, and are often used in conjunction with the modules and other resources.

There has been considerable debate about the need to dissect versus the use of prosections for learning anatomy (Older 2004). Certainly dissection helps a student develop a three-dimensional appreciation of relationships. However, we have found that if a student actively handles and works with prosections, the same understanding can be achieved. The appropriate use of prosections offers several advantages over dissection:

■ Excellent quality specimens can be prepared by a professional dissector. Seldom is the novice student so skilled.

■ A collection of materials can be prepared to best show various structures. During dissection one must choose a particular dissection approach and often one structure must be destroyed in order to visualize another.

■ The collection of prosections can be made available to students so that they can be readily accessed as learner needs dictate.

■ Prosections can be prepared so that they can be palpated or moved, as in the case of joints. The preparation of good quality prosections of joints that can be used for studying movement requires considerable expertise and time. A range of limb prosections, including movable joint specimens, are particularly useful for students who are learning physical assessment.

3

For several years the clinical skills laboratories for the students in the Physiotherapy Program at McMaster University were located in the anatomy laboratory. Linking the learning of anatomy and clinical skills through integrated teaching in a combined resource area provided a stimulating learning environment and greatly enhanced student use of the resources (Groves et al. 1993).

Several years ago an *ultrasound imaging resource* was developed for the anatomy laboratory. The ultrasound machines can be used to view the living body and the movement of structures. Too often students in an anatomy laboratory view internal structures as "fixed" and "rigid." Being able to view the heart valves opening and closing during the cardiac cycle, watching the liver and kidneys move up and down several inches during deep breathing, or observing the flexor tendons and median nerve slide in the carpal tunnel during flexion of the fingers, helps students to better appreciate living anatomy. The proximity of the ultrasound units to the dissected specimens, and other morphology resources, better enables students to integrate their learning (E. Tshibwabwa, personal communication).

More recently there has been an increased focus on using *computer-based resources* to facilitate student learning. Faced with the virtual explosion of learning materials and web sites, it is a challenge to access and evaluate the most valuable sources of information. The resources available in the laboratory include computers with purchased programs, network links, and faculty prepared resources. The location of the computers within the laboratory enables students to readily assess the most appropriate combination of resources to facilitate their learning. Although computers can provide easy access to a large amount of information, they should not be considered a replacement for other resources. Using computers as a replacement for human specimens for learning anatomy has been hotly debated in recent years (Older 2004). Garg et al. (1999) specifically warned that, although digital resources could be valuable enhancements for learning anatomy, they should not be considered superior resources. This is particularly true for students who need to learn through touching and manipulating specimens in order to develop physical assessment skills (Moore 1998). In our experience, the human body is the most important resource for students learning anatomy. It is only through the handling and palpation of specimens that a student can gain a real understanding of three-dimensional structure and its relationship to function.

Strategic organization of the laboratory can facilitate efficient use of the resources. Related resources should be located close together. For example, at McMaster University, upper limb modules and specimens are located together, and adjacent to the lower limb resources. There should be sufficient space for students to work together at a module or with specimens. The areas should be flexible so that movable boards can be used to help students illustrate or organize information, and it should be easy to collect other relevant resources in one area for study and discussion. Computers with resources and internet connections should be readily accessible.

The physical space should also be considered when developing a learning laboratory (Bignell et al. 2001). Good lighting is particularly important when using specimens so that fine structures can be easily seen. Good ventilation is essential if preserved specimens are to be used. Carpeting or acoustical panels can be used to improve the acoustical properties of the space so that a number of groups can work and engage in discussions simultaneously without interfering with each other.

Finally, besides having a role in resource development and curriculum design, faculty with particular expertise can have a critical role as sources of information and as teachers. The various teaching roles for faculty will be discussed in the next section.

Facilitating the Learning of Basic Sciences

Faculty with expertise in a particular discipline can be apprehensive about participation in an integrated program. Their past worth and salaries may have been dependent on their ability to teach didactically in their basic science area of expertise. Participation in an integrated curriculum may place them in a teaching situation where they do not feel competent, while simultaneously removing the confidence they used to feel in their subject area. Careful recruitment of faculty, open discussions of the implication of facilitating learning in an integrated curriculum, and faculty development programs are essential, particularly if transitioning from an established didactic program to a more active learning environment. Friedman et al. (1990) recommended that faculty satisfaction should be assessed when evaluating innovative medical curricula. Once comfortable with innovative programs, faculty do develop satisfaction with PBL or other innovative curricula (Tavanaiepour et al. 2002; Vernon 1995; Vernon and Hosokawa 1996).

Faculty can assume a variety of roles in teaching the basic sciences depending on the philosophy and nature of the program and student needs. In the Physiotherapy and Occupational Therapy Programs at McMaster University, students do not have a formal anatomy or other basic sciences courses (Saarinen and Salvatori 1994). The students are responsible for identifying when they are unable to adequately meet their learning needs through self-directed learning, and when they require additional information. Students may seek additional information from faculty or others with expertise in the area. If a group of students seeking assistance is small, five to seven, all the students in the group are more likely to engage in discussions and ask questions that facilitate their learning. Often a tutorial group will have common learning needs and will request a session as a group, although students also seek individual help.

In other programs, activities such as laboratories, large group sessions, and lectures may be scheduled, or a hybrid of requested and scheduled sessions are used. One of the biggest challenges in providing scheduled sessions for large numbers of students is timing the sessions so that the students encounter the stimulus for learning before the resource session is held. Sequencing and timing are important. If the stimulus to learn does not come first, a student will be less motivated, have done little or no preparation, and will not be ready to learn. If information is given to the students before they have identified a real "need to know and understand," then they are less engaged in the learning process.

When presenting to a large group, it can be a challenge to provide the basic sciences information at a level appropriate for all students. This is particularly true in programs where the educational background and experience of the students entering the program vary widely. For example, students entering the professional training programs in the Faculty of Health Sciences at McMaster University may include students who have graduate degrees in the biological sciences and worked as teaching assistants in gross anatomy or physiology, while other students have expertise in the social sciences with little or no background in biology. Therefore, there may be major differences in levels of knowledge among students, particularly early in their training. With a large group it is challenging for a faculty member to determine the level of the students' knowledge and understanding so that they can tailor their information. Although students may be reluctant to ask questions in a large group, in a small group, particularly with a little encouragement, students are often more willing to question and hypothesize. This can provide faculty with important information that enables

3

them to better targeting of their teaching sessions to meet the learning needs of the students. Questions asked by one student can also have a catalytic effect on discussion and learning for the whole group.

Students who have learned basic sciences in formal structured lectures and laboratories usually feel more secure in this type of learning environment and are often reluctant to adopt a new approach. Students experience stress as they adapt to student-centered curricula (Solomon and Finch 1998). Several strategies can be used to help students to adapt to a new learning environment, to become active learners, and to optimize their learning of the basic sciences content. Most students will become enthusiastic learners if there is a strong stimulus to learn, the resources are informative and exciting to use, and the students can gain a clear understanding of relevant information that satisfies their "need to know."

The strategies for helping students to develop good learning skills for basic sciences are similar to those used for developing learning skills in other areas of the curriculum. Faculty who use and support similar approaches to learning across the curriculum, synergistically foster and facilitate the development of appropriate learning skills. In order to promote independent learning, students need to become familiar with the types of resources that can be used to meet their learning needs, and they need to be able to access and use those resources efficiently and effectively (Greening 1998). Some students may not be comfortable using particular resources, such as a human anatomy laboratory, and may need assistance to learn how to best use these resources.

For a student to develop learning skills, it is important that they understand how they learn. A common question from students starting to learn in the anatomy laboratory is "What is the best way to learn anatomy?" When the response is "How do you learn best?", it is frequently surprising to find that many students have little understanding of their own learning strengths or weaknesses. Is the student a visual, auditory, or tactile learner, or do they use these approaches in various combinations (Rose 1985)? Some are very strong in one area and particularly weak in another. It is useful for students to determine the strategies that work best for them. Students may need assistance, and even some persuasion, to develop these skills.

Special Issues for Facilitating the Learning of Anatomy

The study of anatomy is required in a number of educational programs, in-depth knowledge and understanding of functional morphology being a requirement of many of these programs. Faculty have several roles in facilitating the learning of anatomy in an integrated curriculum. They ensure that appropriate stimuli are embedded in the curriculum, that students develop the appropriate learning skills unique to anatomy, and that they stimulate and support active learning of relevant information. In addition, faculty face the challenge of helping new students adjust to working with human material and learning in the laboratory setting.

The *orientation* to the anatomy laboratory is important as it sets the context and tone for future learning. Although most students approach an anatomy laboratory for the first time with a sense of excitement and enthusiasm that enables them to quickly become engaged learners, a surprising number of students experience a degree of anxiety. In some cases this can be severe and markedly effect their ability to learn (Dickinson et al. 1997; Evans and Fitzgibbon 1992). Since most of these students are reluctant to admit they are uncomfortable, often their concerns are not addressed. Thus, it is important to introduce new students to the laboratory in a manner that helps them become more comfortable working and learning in this environment. There are several strategies that can be used to help the students. Since working directly with specimens or dissecting a body generates the greatest apprehension, overcoming anxiety and replacing it with a level of comfort and enthusiasm for learning presents a challenge. Since anxiety often grows with anticipation, it is useful to introduce students to using specimens early on, preferably during the first visit to the anatomy laboratory. They tend to be less anxious if they are in small groups where they can share the experience and provide support for each other. A specimen that is small and interesting tends to be less threatening than a whole body or limb.

The following approach is used for anatomy laboratory orientation for students in rehabilitation sciences at McMaster University. Students are asked to consider how they use their elbow to carry out particular tasks such as eating a cookie or opening a door. Once students feel and observe these movements at their own elbow, they are given articulated bones to move and observe. Since students are seldom uncomfortable working with the bones, it is usually easy to get them engaged in handling and discussing the material. Simultaneously moving and examining one's own elbow or that of a partner, helps students relate the skeletal material to living functional anatomy, and can be used to start students thinking about the muscles responsible for moving the joint. This sets the stage for the transition to examining dissected "wet" specimens. A deeply dissected small specimen of the elbow is a wet specimen, but it does not tend to be intimidating because it is similar to the bones the students are familiar with yet it provides additional information relevant to muscles and movements. Appropriate questions stimulate discussion of the new learning and its application. At this point, students who were apprehensive coming into the laboratory, and who were at risk of becoming increasingly anxious, are usually more comfortable and better prepared to start learning.

Providing a good orientation to learning in a human anatomy laboratory provides an important foundation for the students' future learning. At McMaster University, we have found that senior students can assist in the orientation process and serve as role models for the new students. Second-year medical and rehabilitation sciences students assist faculty in the orientation of the new students. They take small groups through the laboratory, stimulate discussion of resources and how these are used to facilitate learning, and provide support and encouragement.

The next challenge is to help students become enthusiastic active learners. Unfortunately anatomy has a reputation as a subject with a huge amount of terminology that requires memorization. This can appear overwhelming to a new student. Initially it may be useful to use common terms in parallel with anatomical terms in order to get students engaged in learning and discussion, without becoming overwhelmed. Saying that a particular muscle "lies closer to the middle or more medial" or "when the hand is pronated or turned so the palm faces down," allows the novice to understand and participate in discussions. Students will quickly adopt the anatomical and clinical terminology as their knowledge and confidence increases, and as they apply their learning in other areas of the curriculum. This also provides the opportunity to help students recognize that most anatomical terms are related to structure and function. One could pose the question "if the *flexor carpi ulnaris* lies on the ulnar side of the arm, crosses carpal bones and flexes the wrist, then what would you call a similar muscle that inserts on the radial side?" This approach focuses on developing understanding rather than on the isolated memorization of names.

In our experience, faculty also have an important role in helping students develop the observational and reasoning skills that are particularly important for learning human anatomy. Asking basic questions in the anatomy laboratory such as, "What are your learning objectives?", "What do you think this is and what is its function?", or "How do you think it might be injured and how would function be affected?", challenge students to observe, hypothesize, develop reasoning skills, and consider how they can apply the information while they are working with the specimens. This not only enhances the learning of anatomy, but also facilitates the integration of the information. A faculty member with specific expertise can help guide student learning or provide information when appropriate. As their learning skills develop, students become increasingly efficient and capable of more independent learning.

The following is an example of a problem that could be used to stimulate learning about the functional anatomy of the hand:

> *Mrs. Simpson, a 36-year-old computer programmer, complains of numbness, tingling, and pain in her right hand. She notes that her little finger seems "okay". Symptoms, which began several years ago, were mild at first but became progressively worse since she became pregnant.*
>
> This problem should stimulate students to learn about the functional anatomy of the hand and, specifically, the structures that are involved in producing the described symptoms. In the anatomy laboratory students can examine specimens of the hand and carpal tunnel. The structures that form the tunnel and its contents, including the tendons and median nerve, can be examined and identified. They can appreciate the small size of the tunnel and note that its dimensions are decreased during wrist flexion or extension, as often occurs when using a keyboard, and increased when the wrist is in a "neutral" position. A well-prepared specimen can enable the students to identify and follow the sensory branches of the median nerve that serve the same area that is affected by the sensory changes noted by Mrs. Simpson. The muscles innervated by the median nerve can also be examined, and the effects on hand motor function of prolonged compression resulting in median nerve damage discussed. The possible association between symptoms and increased water retention in pregnancy might also be considered.

A problem such as this should stimulate students to develop an understanding of the functional anatomy relevant to the cause of the problem, the symptoms, the possible complications, and strategies for treatment.

Evaluation of Basic Sciences Knowledge

Since reward reinforces behavior and evaluation drives learning (Grand'Maison et al. 2002; Williams et al. 2003), students tend to invest their efforts in those activities that provide them with the best reward or highest mark. To support and reinforce the desired approach to learning basic sciences, it is important that the methods used for evaluating knowledge reward both the acquisition of content and the curricular approach. For example, if students using a problem-based approach are expected to identify learning objectives, acquire a detailed knowledge and understanding of the topic, and apply the information to the problem, then it is important to use methods of evaluation that not only determine their basic sciences content knowledge, but also assess their ability to reason and apply this knowledge. If students are tested only on their content knowledge, then they are likely to focus their efforts on gathering facts rather than on developing a deeper understanding of information. If students are asked to identify structures in an anatomy examination and there is no evaluation of their understanding of function or its clinical importance, even students that have been involved in PBL may tend to revert to memorizing facts rather that gaining a more in-depth understanding of functional morphology. Morrison and Murray (1994 p. 145) stated that "By the time the students enter the final rotation of their medical course they are already preoccupied with passing their final examinations. As their course so far has tended to encourage superficial learning likely to aid in passing examinations, the problem-based learning, which was felt to be time-consuming although promoting deep learning…was judged to be less relevant."

There is evidence that evaluation of knowledge and its application enhances learning of basic sciences content in PBL curricula (Sivam et al. 1995; Sweeney 1999). There are two general approaches that may be useful for evaluating a student's basic sciences knowledge and understanding that can also help to reinforce integrated learning. One approach is to incorporate basic sciences content questions into applied or practical evaluations such as objective structured clinical evaluations (OCSEs) or modified essay questions. For example, at an OSCE station where students are asked to evaluate the strength of the muscles that extend the knee, they could also be asked to identify the nerve that innervates the muscles or the processes involved in muscle contraction. Alternatively, applied or reasoning questions can be incorporated into the stations in an anatomy "bell-ringer" examination. Rather than just asking for the origin, insertion, and innervation of a muscle, one could include questions on function of the muscle, possible mechanisms for injuring a particular nerve, or the effects of the injury on function. In this way, evaluation not only serves to test a student's knowledge, but also influences the student's approach to learning.

Conclusion

Integrating the basic sciences into innovative curricula presents a number of challenges, while offering unique opportunities and significant rewards. The challenges include determining the important content that is needed and deciding on the most effective strategies for incorporating the content into the curriculum. Appropriate resources need to be available to support good learning. Although resources could include an extensive collection of materials in a large laboratory and state of the art computer-based resources, other resources such as those prepared by faculty or sought out by the students can also support excellent learning. For students with a traditional educational background, who are not familiar with innovative approaches to learning, faculty members play a critical role in fostering the development of learning skills and facilitating the appropriate use of resources.

An innovative curriculum with integrated basic sciences provides students with a stimulating and engaging opportunity for excellence in learning. The desire to learn and understand the subject can be compelling, the knowledge valued and its application appreciated. Evaluation should be designed to reinforce integrated learning.

References

Barrows HS, Tamblyn RM (1980) Problem-based learning: an approach to medical education. Springer, Berlin Heidelberg New York (Medical education, vol 1)

Bignell J, Groves H, Bayley L (2001) Developing learning and library resources. In: Rideout E (ed) Transforming nursing education through problem-based learning. Jones and Bartlett, Sudbury, MA

Blake J (1994) Library resources for problem-based learning: the program perspective. Comput Methods Programs Biomed 44:167–173

Coles CR (1985) Differences between conventional and problem-based curricula in their students' approach to studying. Med Educ 9:308–309

Dangerfield P, Bradley P, Gibbs T (2000) Learning gross anatomy in a clinical skills course. Clin Anat 13:444–447

Dickinson GE, Lancaster CJ, Winfield IE, Reece EF, Colthorpe CA (1997) Detached concern and death anxiety of first-year medical students: before and after the gross anatomy course. Clin Anat 10:201–207

Evans EJ, Fitzgibbon GH (1992) The dissecting room: reactions of first year medical students. Clin Anat 5:311–320

Friedman CP, de Blick R, Greer DS, Mennin SP, Norman GR, Sheps CG, Swanson DB, Woodward CA (1990) Charting the winds of change: evaluating innovative medical curricula. Acad Med 65:8–14

Gardner H (1993) Frames of mind: the theory of multiple intelligences, 10th anniversary edn. Basic Books, New York, NY

Garg A, Norman GR, Spero L, Maheshwari P (1999) Do virtual computer models hinder anatomy learning? Acad Med 74:587–589

Grand'Maison P, Brailovsky C, Emond J-G (2002) Evaluation drives learning: is this true for a performance-based licensing examination? Canadian Association of Medical Education, Research and Development Abstracts. http://www.came-acem.ca/Pages/Meeting-2002AbstractsR&D.html

Greening T (1998) Scaffolding for success in PBL. Med Educ Online (serial online) 3,4. Available from http://www.Med-Ed-Online.org

Groves H, Crowe J, Stratford P, Binkley J (1993) Clinical skills in the anatomy laboratory: linking the learning. Programme of the international conference on student centred education in conjunction with the 8th biennial general network meeting, Sherbrooke, Canada, 22–27 August 1993, p 145

Kolb DA (1984) Experiential learning: experience as the source of learning and development. Prentice-Hall, Englewood Cliffs, NJ

MacLeod SM (1999) Basic sciences in medical education. Clin Invest Med 22:23–24

Marshall JG, Fitzgerald D, Busby L, Heaton G (1993) A study of library use in problem-based and traditional medical curricula. Bull Med Libr Assoc 81:299–305

Mizer LA, Farnum CE, Schenck PD (2002) The modular resource centre: integrating units for the study of the anatomical sciences in a problem-based curriculum. Anat Rec 269:249–256

Moore NA (1998) To dissect or not to dissect? Anat Rec 253:8–9

Morrison JM, Murray TS (1994) An experiment in problem-based learning. Med Educ 28:139–145

Newble DI, Clarke RM (1986) The approaches to learning of students in a traditional and in an innovative problem-based medical school. Acad Med 67:557–565

Older J (2004) Matter for debate: anatomy: a must for teaching the next generation. Surg J R Coll Surg Edinb Irel 2:79–90

Pallie W, Brain E (1978) 'Modules' in morphology for self study: a system for learning in an undergraduate medical programme. Med Educ 12:107–113

Pallie W, Carr DH (1987) The McMaster medical education philosophy in theory, practise and historical perspective. Med Teach 9:59–71

Pallie W, Miller D (1982) Communicating morphology concepts in health sciences. J Biocommun 9:26–32

Prince KJ, van Maneren H, Hylkema N, Drukker J, Scherpbier AJ, van der Veluten CP (2003) Does problem-based learning lead to deficiencies in basic sciences knowledge? An empirical case on anatomy. Med Educ 37:15–21

Rangachari PK (1997) Basic sciences in an integrated medical curriculum: the case of pharmacology. Adv Health Sci Educ 2:163–171

Rose C (1985) Accelerated learning. Dell, New York, NY

Saarinen H, Salvatori P (1994) Dialogue: educating occupational and physiotherapists for the year 2000: what, no anatomy courses? Physiother Can 46:81–86

Sivam SP, Iatridis PG, Vaughn S (1995) Integration of pharmacology into a problem-based learning curriculum for medical students. Med Educ 29:289–296

Smith DM, Kolb DA (1986) The user's guide for the learning-style inventory: a manual for teachers and trainers. McBer, Boston, MA

Solomon P, Finch E (1998) A qualitative study identifying stressors associated with adapting to problem-based learning. Teach Learn Med 10:58–64

Sweeney G (1999) The challenge for basic science education in problem-based medical curricula. Clin Invest Med 22:15–22

Tavanaiepour D, Schwartz PL, Loten EG (2002) Faculty opinions about a revised pre-clinical curriculum. Med Educ 36:299–302

Vernon DTA (1995) Attitudes and opinions of faculty tutors about problem-based learning. Acad Med 70:216–223

Vernon DTA, Hosokawa MC (1996) Faculty attitudes and opinions about problem-based learning. Acad Med 71:1233–1238

Williams R, MacDermid J, Wessel J (2003) Student adaptation to problem-based learning in an entry-level master's physical therapy program. Physiother Theory Pract 19:119–212

Zehr CL, Butler RG, Richardson R J (1996) Students' use of anatomy modules in problem-based medical education at McMaster University. Acad Med 71:1015–1017

Chapter 4

Developing Emerging Roles in Clinical Education

4

Bonny Jung, Patricia Solomon, Beverley Cole

>> Fieldwork education needs to constantly evolve through a process
of development and evaluation of new initiatives.
(Prigg and Mackenzie 2000)

Since the mid-1990s, a number of factors have impacted on the way clinical education
has been conceptualized and implemented. In planning innovative curricula, educators must consider issues such as available resources within the clinical and university
sectors, credentialing changes, educational advances and initiatives, increased enrolment within the universities, and role innovations and development within professional practice. These factors have all contributed to the need to rethink and re-exam-
ine ways of doing things. hooks (1994 p. 207) speaks of the learning environment as,
"…a location of possibility. In that field of possibility we have the opportunity to labor
for freedom, to demand of ourselves…an openness of mind and heart that allows us to
face reality even as we collectively imagine ways to move beyond boundaries, to transgress. This is education as the practice of freedom." This is not to say that we should be
creating placement experiences with no structure and unlimited amounts of freedom!
Van Manen (2002 p. 62) identifies the learner as needing "…controlled freedom as well
as control that pushes freedom forward." Cranton (1992 p. 106) states, "being a self-directed learner is a freeing experience. The very nature of learning changes from trying
to figure out what the teacher wants and repeating it, to exploring, growing, and break-
ing free of boundaries." Cranton identifies the process of self-directed learning as involving phases of transition for the learner that can include: introduction and reactions to the new way of learning; renewed interest and excitement; reorientation; equi-
librium; and finally advocacy.

Implementation of innovative placements that facilitate emerging roles may be
easier in student-centered curricula that allow students to determine and pursue their
own learning needs and objectives. Students are given some power in the direction of
their learning and the way they can learn. Problem-based learning (PBL) provides an
ideal context for students to create spaces for discourse and practice within boundaries that support and protect rather than bind and restrict. This style of learning creates
an environment whereby the learner can enter into self-reflection in dealing with the
demands of their ideals and the demands of reality. In doing so, the learner can find
new views that can ultimately contribute to her/his understanding of self and of the
profession.

Across the health care disciplines, many terms have been used to describe the clinical learning experience and stakeholders involved in clinical fieldwork education. In
this chapter, the terms "preceptor" will be used when referring to the clinical supervis-
or, "placement" when referring to the student fieldwork experience, "site" when referring to the agency or organization providing the placement, and "clinical education"
when referring to the educational curricular program. Although there is an abundance
of literature across disciplines related to clinical education, we have chosen to focus
primarily on the findings from physiotherapy and occupational therapy. This chapter
will review issues related to clinical education, the status of role-emerging placements
within occupational therapy and physiotherapy, provide illustrative examples, and
highlight some lessons learned through our experiences. We begin some of the following sections with a quote from a student who had participated in a role-emerging
placement.

Need for Innovations in Clinical Education

> ❯❯ So it came alive, a lot of those skills that we really needed to use, the skills that you learned somewhat artificially in school.

Clinical education constitutes a significant portion of the students' educational program in the rehabilitation sciences, and is a key component in the preparation of competent physiotherapists and occupational therapists (Deusinger 1990; Tompson and Proctor 1990). Cohn and Crist (1995) see clinical education as the essential bridge from the classroom to the practice setting whereby the supervising therapist or preceptor plays a leading role in shaping the future of the profession.

Most placements involve the assignment of a student or students to a therapist within a setting in which the therapist has a defined role. Placements can utilize different models of learning and/or supervision of which the advantages and disadvantages have been well documented in the literature. Some reported models of clinical education include one student to two therapists (Gaiptman and Forma 1991), part-time therapist to full-time student (Desrosiers et al. 1997), two students to one therapist (Ladyshewsky 1995; Solomon and Sanford 1993; Tiberious and Gaiptman 1985), student peer supervision (Bossers et al. 1997b), and cooperative, collaborative or group (Declute and Ladyshewsky 1993; Farrow et al. 2000; Jung et al. 1994; Mason 1998). Hamlin et al. (1995) also raise the possibility of reconceptualizing the foundations of clinical education. They suggest exploring and developing placement settings in light of the domains of learning they can offer. This method of description would allow recognition of a more holistic view of the clients and setting and potentially facilitate the numbers of placements available for students.

Historically physiotherapists and occupational therapists received the bulk of their clinical education in hospital or institutional settings. As the professions matured and moved to community settings and towards more consultative roles, there has been an increased need for clinical education experiences in these areas of practice. However, the shift in practice settings in conjunction with the constraints of limited time and increased workload (Canadian Association of Occupational Therapy [CAOT] 1991; Green 1996; Hurley 2000; Sloggett et al. 2003; Tompson and Proctor 1990) have posed barriers to offering placements. In Canada, many physiotherapy and occupational therapy programs report an ongoing shortage of clinical placements (CAOT 1991; Council of Ontario Universities 2004). Backman (1994) stated that there are no shortages of learning opportunities. She noted that every placement was a perfect placement, that we need to "stop obsessing over the details thought to contribute to the perfect placement" (Backman 1994 p. 9), and that core skills can be learned in many areas beyond direct, therapeutic client care activities. Aiken et al. (2001) suggest that clinical education must reflect current contexts and trends of health/community care and that no recipe exists for the ideal format and content of this component of the curriculum. The reality of health care is that therapists frequently find themselves working in areas where they have no immediate director or supervisor and must practice autonomously with limited supervision (Westmorland and Jung 1997) and guideline protocols. This is true even of new graduates (Miller et al. 2002).

The reported placement shortages have prompted educators to continue to develop innovative placement experiences. However, the advantages of developing a new and emerging area of practice go far beyond providing additional clinical sites for a university program. Students are often provided with opportunities to learn consultation skills, to engage in program development and evaluation, and to educate others about the role of occupational therapy and physiotherapy. Through working independently and advocating for their professional role, students learn skills that will serve them well as they enter the profession.

What Is the Role-emerging Placement?

The majority of literature in the area of role-emerging placements has appeared in the occupational therapy literature. "Role-emerging" is a relatively new term used to describe a placement in a setting that does not have an established program or a staff person hired to fulfill the role, is coordinated and supervised by an off-site licensed therapist who is not employed by the setting, and the student is assigned to a site staff person as a contact for site concerns (Bossers et al. 1997a). Other authors in occupational therapy have described similar models using different terminology. Heubner and Tryssenaar (1996) refer to a homeless shelter placement as "non-traditional," Westmorland and Jung (1997) refer to a food processing plant placement as "creative and innovative," and Alsop and Donald (1996) refer to the term "atypical." Additionally, Prigg and Mackenzie (2000) developed the "project" placement that has similar characteristics to the role-emerging placement. In the project placement, community sites initiated projects based on their organizational needs and students were expected to work independently and cooperatively with another student under minimal supervision.

Regulatory requirements for direct on-site supervision of students have hindered the development of role-emerging placements in physiotherapy. Much of the literature has focused on the unique and innovative roles that physiotherapists are developing with new conditions and in different types of settings. For example, Benson et al. (1995) described the role of the army physiotherapist as a non-physician health care provider who could prescribe certain medications. Nixon and Cott (2000) reconceptualized human immunodeficiency virus (HIV) disease within a rehabilitation framework, outlining the potential of physiotherapeutic interventions for people living with HIV. Several authors have investigated the emerging role of the physiotherapist in neuropsychiatry and psychiatry (Behr and Brunham 2002; Maestri 1996). Others have advocated for a conceptual role shift within the more traditional hospital setting (Taylor et al. 1997). While this literature illustrates exciting new opportunities for physiotherapists, typically clinical education is not a component in the evolution of the emerging role. In a synthesis of the physiotherapy clinical education literature, Strohschein et al. (2002) described various models and tools that currently exist to guide the general process. Of these, the role-emerging placement is not identified; however, these authors do propose that a combination of qualitative, descriptive, and experimental research can illuminate the multidimensional nature of the process. These findings can subsequently assist physiotherapists in selecting the appropriate and available models and/or to develop new models that can address the unique needs of physiotherapy clinical education.

What Are the Benefits?

》 It seemed overwhelming at first, but after some digestion, I have identified some learning issues. This may include negotiating, compromising, and most of all communicating with all the stakeholders…skills that can be enhanced and implemented into every interpersonal relationship – professional or otherwise. This will not be a "traditional" placement by any means, but an opportunity to gains skills in many new areas.

The benefits of role-emerging placements for both the student and the site have been widely discussed. Bossers et al. (1997a) found four key student benefits: (1) learning to view the client as a person rather than focusing on the diagnosis; (2) experiencing personal growth with increased compassion; (3) a greater comfort level in working with clients; and (4) engaging in a variety of new and expanded roles that were different from those experienced within more typical hierarchically organized institutions. Factors that contributed to the learning experience were the community context, placement structure, pre-placement preparation, and consultation model of supervision. They summarized, the "role-emerging placement is a valuable, viable model of fieldwork and needs to be recognized as legitimate and even preferred for some of the types of learning that may happen more readily through its role-creation structure" (Bossers et al. 1997a p. 79).

Soltys et al. (1997) highlighted the need for the role-emerging placement to be a controlled, yet well-supervised learning experience. They described important learning outcomes such as greater opportunities to understand the roles of other disciplines and for other disciplines to learn about occupational therapy; increased understanding of the role of the occupational therapist as a consultant; greater confidence in problem-solving; increased flexibility and ability to prioritize decisions; and enhanced professional identity. Role-emerging placements have also been reported to give students, educational programs, and the sites, opportunities to widen horizons, to venture into new situations, and to do cutting edge work (Alsop and Donald 1996; Pontello and Tryssenaar 1996). Pontello and Tryssenaar (1996) added that the student–preceptor relationship should be collegial and flexible, fostering mutual reflective speculation. Building trust between the student and preceptor is a primary and key element in this relationship. Huebner and Tryssenaar (1996) found, in a role-emerging shelter placement, that placements do not need to be all about physical doing. The essentialness of rapport building between the student and client was highlighted. We have observed that many of our students attended to developing, fostering, and maintaining relationships more so in a role-emerging placement than in a traditional placement in order to gain trust with the clients and staff.

With respect to site benefits, Westmorland and Jung (1997) and Wilkins and Jung (2001) described expert services gained through student and faculty that incorporated consultation on the management of specific health conditions, staff education through provision of research articles and resources and workshops, and initiation of program evaluation methods. We have also found other site benefits such as increased staff familiarity with the professional role, development of future employment opportunities, and initiation of collaborative site/university research projects.

In the area of interdisciplinary learning, Miller and Ishler (2001) discussed the benefits of a model for team training in a clinical learning experience. Occupational therapy, physiotherapy, physician assistant, and public health students were supported and supervised by their school faculty as they participated in a non-traditional placement project that provided service to rural, community-dwelling older adults. The students identified positive outcomes such as gaining interdisciplinary team knowledge and skills, and direct client contact. This is also consistent with the findings from Solomon et al. (2003) that paired physiotherapy and occupational students in role-emerging placements in a community health care center, servicing clients with HIV.

In summary, role-emerging placements offer significant benefits to both the student and the site. The educational program is able to expand pedagogical principles into new sites of learning, increase the base of placement opportunities, work effectively within available resources, and develop and expand present and future roles.

What Are the Challenges?

> I think you need to have a certain personality to go into an emerging role…the flexibility, the strong goal setting, problem-solving and really willing to branch out…someone who is willing to take that step and is willing to make a mistake and willing to not have things work out the way you would like.

We have found that many students, when choosing their placements, opt for the hospital setting as these are perceived to be more established and often have links with teaching universities. Also, these sites are in well-known institutions and located in major centers and therefore are also more geographically desirable. Most students enter educational programs with a preconceived or limited impression of what a therapist does and where they work and are truly surprised with the different array of possibilities. When starting a community placement setting, students might have the curative, medical model foremost in their mind, which may influence how adaptable they are to the setting (Solomon and Sanford 1993). They may also be concerned if they perceive that their placements do not allow them to practice "traditional" hands-on skills. In our experience this has been exacerbated in physiotherapy since the introduction of a national licensing examination with a clinical skills evaluation component. Bilics et al. (2002) found that students consistently expressed anxiety during the initial stages of the placement, questioning their understanding of the role and their knowledge of appropriate client intervention programs. However, as the students progressed through the experience, they began to realize that they do have these skills and could see themselves practicing in non-traditional areas in the future. This transition is consistent with Cranton's (1992) view of possible learner reactions in working towards self-directed learning.

Prigg and Mackenzie (2000) found that there was a difference in perception of the clinical education experience between the student and preceptor following a role-emerging placement. The preceptors expressed more positive feedback about the student placement experience than that given by the students. Prigg and Mackenzie felt that this might have been due to the decreased face-to-face contact time with the students, and thereby the supervisors might have been less aware of the students' perceptions. Decreased face-to-face contact time is common to role-emerging placements that utilize two students to one therapist and group supervision models. The limited direct contact time between the student and the preceptor requires that the student work with some degree of autonomy and independence. In placements of short duration (i.e., 5–6 weeks), there may be insufficient time for full development of the student roles with the clients and the setting, or for other team members to become familiar with student roles (Solomon et al. 2003). Many of our students report that they need more up front time to get their bearings, identify the resources, develop clearer objectives, and implement the plan of action. One student exclaimed, "by the time you figure out what you are doing, it's over!" Often, students and their preceptors need to go back to the basics and ask questions such as, "what is the role of the OT/PT in health care?", "what is the role of the OT/PT in this setting?", and "what can I offer that meets the specific needs of this community?".

Another quandary for educators is determining whether it is better to offer role-emerging placements to students in the early or later phases of their professional education. Bossers et al. (1997a) suggest that role-emerging placements are suitable for a student's senior placement. Based on our experiences, given careful planning, both junior and senior students can benefit from these learning experiences.

A common challenge we have encountered when organizing a placement without an on-site therapist is recruiting a knowledgeable preceptor who is comfortable with the supervision model and able to access the site throughout the placement. In the past, clinicians who have clinical faculty appointments played this role. One solution is having the site provide funds to hire a preceptor; however, many sites have limited resources. Another option is that faculty can provide supervision. Etcheverry (1994) notes that faculty liaison plays an important role in facilitating student learning, assisting with problem resolution, and developing communication links between academics and clinicians. Despite the recognized benefits of faculty involvement at the more direct supervision level, this can still be a challenge for faculty with heavy educational and research commitments. Extensive planning is required to develop a role-emerging placement. Identifying and negotiating with sites to develop the placement, as well as integrating the experiences into courses that support the placement, is extremely time consuming (Bilics et al. 2002). Sullivan and Finlayson (2000) established a university-funded, contract position for a role-emerging project coordinator to develop, negotiate, and adequately supervise role-emerging placements as an added resource to the university faculty.

Liability can be a concern for the site and the preceptor. Some settings prefer not to have an affiliation agreement addressing the legal responsibilities; however, most universities require a formal agreement before students are placed in any setting. These agreements can be daunting at the best of times! Working with the administration and human resource staff requires careful collaboration. It may take many revisions before all parties are satisfied. There may be times when the concerns cannot be reconciled between organizations despite the support from the preceptor and the immediate site representative. Some of our placements have been canceled primarily due to the inability to work out a mutually satisfactory affiliation agreement. Preceptors may also be apprehensive about being responsible for a student they will not be seeing regularly. Regulatory bodies have guidelines that address student supervision; however, they can be perceived as restrictive rather than supportive. In the study by Wilkins and Jung (2002), the student's direct client interventions were modified because of preceptor concerns about accountability and liability.

These innovative placement experiences, despite the challenges, encompass the notions of moving beyond the boundaries, entering new terrains of experiences and learning, and developing and enhancing new and different relationships. In doing so, mutually beneficial partnerships are forged between the stakeholders.

In order to formulate a shift from the theoretical and conceptual to the practical, we have provided three examples in Appendix 1 based on our experiences that illustrate some of the applied concepts related to role-emerging placements. They are presented in ways that highlight different issues as we have found that each experience teaches us something unique.

Lessons Learned

4

Through our experiences at McMaster University we have found several strategies that facilitate success in role-emerging placements. These can be adapted to suit institutional requirements related to academic accreditation and regulatory body standards, educational program pedagogy, community needs, student objectives, and resources available.

1. Attend to pre-placement planning and orientation

   Pre-placement preparation is crucial to the success of any placement and for the role-emerging experience this is particularly so. Engaging the stakeholders early in the planning and development process promotes a collaborative approach. Given that the student is placed in a setting that does not have a defined role, both the student and the preceptor will need to work together to research the clinical evidence, apply theory to practice, and problem-solve through new situations as they explore the potential professional roles and responsibilities. At McMaster University we have found that it is not unusual to explore the placement site a few years in advance. The site requires time to consider the proposal, plan for the educational experience, and ensure that administrative matters are in order. A sample proposal included in Appendix 2 provides a framework for developing a correspondence. Developing affiliation agreements and sorting out the liability concerns require patience and ongoing negotiation and communication. Additionally the site may want their program to be at a certain level of maturity and stability before offering the educational experience. It is important to understand that the present time may not be the right time for the site and to respect their participation timelines. Be patient and keep the door open for future connections.

2. Establish clear yet flexible expectations/objectives

   As with any placement, clear student objectives must be established; however, it is important to have a degree of flexibility in the expected outcomes. Since the role is not clearly delineated, the student will be testing new concepts and strategies. The objectives should be used as outcomes to work towards but should not be so restricting that they limit and demobilize the student from action. We want to foster the curiosity and enthusiasm that occur when the student is faced with a new and unique situation. Innovations usually are initiated through acting on those student queries and subsequently stretching the boundaries of practice.

3. Consider alternative teaching–learning strategies

   In a traditional, role-established setting, the preceptor has many opportunities to use direct observation to assess student learning. Also, the student is able to readily connect with the preceptor or other therapists within the setting for advice and consultation. Given that this type of contact is not always available, alternative methods of teaching and learning can facilitate learning. An interactive journal is an excellent tool that can encourage self-reflection and clinical reasoning (Jensen and Denton 1991; Perkins 1996; Tryssenaar 1994). When using journals, it is helpful to discuss issues such as the purpose (teaching and/or evaluation), confidentiality considerations (who will read it), and expected frequency (how often submitted). A sample journal may be helpful for those who are unfamiliar with the process and format. Communication among all stakeholders is critical to clarify the expectations and learning processes. When face-to-face meetings are not possible, or are limited, strategies for distance supervision can include telephone and email contacts and videoconferencing (Sullivan and Finlayson 2000). It is important to have the communication schedule and preferred strategies arranged at the beginning of the placement.

4. Foster a trusting and open student–preceptor relationship

Students may find that they are in situations of ambiguity and uncertainty. It is critical that they feel comfortable expressing their anxieties and concerns to the preceptor, which will happen only if a positive trusting relationship is established early. Students need to know that they are in a safe and supportive learning environment. Some thought and consideration needs to be put into the selection of the preceptor and student. We have found that a preceptor who is comfortable with the concepts of "managing" the caseload differently and "trusting" the student adapts better to these kinds of placements. Cranton (1992) suggests that to be successful in implementing self-directed learning, the educator should truly believe in the learners' ability to direct their own learning and to be able to give up responsibility to learners when it is appropriate. The preceptor will rely primarily on feedback from the student, the on-site resource person, and other team members to develop appropriate client profiles and to formulate a judgment of the student's performance. Not all preceptors feel comfortable with this type of arrangement. The preceptor who possesses characteristics that encompass skills in self-direction, critical thinking, self-reflection, communication, and professionalism will be ideal.

The key characteristics that we look for in a student are motivation to learn, ability to self-reflect, and willingness to take risks. It is critical that the student has choice in selecting this type of placement so that it fits with her/his own interest and preferences. Assigning a student who is not interested can only result in disappointment and/or failure. Sullivan and Finlayson (2000) developed guidelines to facilitate student selection and student engagement in the process that considered student self-selection, a student-written report of preferences and integration into professional practice, and evaluation of the student's abilities and insights by the role-emerging project coordinator.

5. Pair/group students and encourage student support network

Assigning students in pairs or in a small group in a role-emerging placement provides opportunities for peer teaching and problem-solving to occur. Additionally students can provide immediate support to each other on matters relating to day-to-day events. Tiberius and Gaiptman (1985) found that one important benefit of pairing students in placement was the decrease in the amount of superficial questions asked by students. We have had successful experiences using a group supervision model in which three or four students are assigned to role-emerging placements. Student support can also be facilitated through internet discussions amongst other students who are in role-emerging placements. They may be able to share stories and solutions to dilemmas faced in their settings.

6. Post-placement synthesis and debriefing

After the placement is over, some students may still be unclear about how to integrate what they have learned into their overall understanding of the profession. At this point, it is important to help the student assess the learning outcomes within the context to her/his profession at a more global level. This can be done by having a debriefing meeting with the student or with the group of students who participated in similar placements within the same block of time. Also, tracking the student over the course of subsequent placements is critical. Sometimes the pieces of the puzzle come together forming a picture only at the end of the educational program.

7. Expect the unexpected

   No matter how well things are planned, be prepared for the unexpected! The blueprint is established for the experience; however, you never really know how it will unfold. Everyone is living the experience for the first time.

4

And lastly, the planning guide in Appendix 3 may be helpful to conceptualize the steps involved in developing, organizing, and implementing the role-emerging placement.

Conclusion

Chomsky (2000) states that education can either be a process of indoctrination or it can provide people with knowledge and skills to develop their critical thinking skills. The role-emerging placement creates spaces where students can strive towards becoming critical thinkers. These placements should be considered an essential part of the "mainstream" curriculum. The issue becomes not whether the placement is in a role-established or role-emerging setting; rather the issue is how we can create enduring and sustaining educational experiences that promote critical thinking regardless of the structure or location. Parker Palmer, as cited in hooks (2003), believes that enlightened teaching evokes and invites community as they are places of source for hope, and where the passion to connect and learn is constantly fulfilled. Palmer adds "...great teaching is about knowing that community, feeling that community, sensing that community and then drawing our students into it" (hooks 2003 p. xvi). Role-emerging placement opportunities facilitate a different way of seeing the world. The students can see past the boundaries of the past and present, and gain flight by acting on possibilities.

Appendix 1

Examples of Interprofessional Placements

1. The Community Health Center Servicing Individuals with HIV

Rationale for Pursuing Placement

Due to advances in pharmacological management, people with HIV are now living longer. In industrialized nations, the natural history of HIV has changed from one of being a terminal illness to one of a chronic, episodic illness. As a result, people with HIV are now living with a variety of impairments and activity limitations that are amenable to rehabilitation efforts. Consequently there is a greater role for rehabilitation, though this is not a well-developed area of expertise for occupational therapy or physiotherapy.

Description of the Placement

A local community health center had an HIV program; however, there were no coordinated rehabilitation services. While two physiotherapists were employed at the center, they were not directly involved in the HIV program. There was no occupational therapist employed at the center. Recognizing the important role for rehabilitation services with clients with HIV at this site, a faculty member approached the site representatives about the possibility of providing interprofessional role-emerging placements for an occupational therapy student and a physiotherapy student. Two senior students who were interested in HIV and had demonstrated superior communication skills in previous placements and the ability to work collaboratively without direct supervision were selected for a 5-week full-time clinical placement. The two staff physiotherapists provided on-site supervision, while occupational and physiotherapy faculty provided off-site consultation and support. In addition to addressing curricular learning objectives, each student developed a learning contract that was specific to the clinical placement.

Unique Accomplishments During the Placement

The students determined that there was a need to develop a joint assessment form for the HIV clients, which focused on assessment of function and incorporated the Canadian Occupational Performance Measure (Law et al. 1998). As part of the overall assessment, the students included a needs-based assessment to determine what services would best meet the needs of HIV clients in the community. Students invited all HIV-positive clients who were registered at the clinic to participate in an initial assessment. From the needs assessment the students determined there were two key areas in which clients living with HIV required additional information: fatigue and pain. Using client education principles addressed during their academic studies, the students developed two educational booklets which provided strategies for self-management of pain and fatigue. Students also presented the findings of their needs assessment to staff at the community health center in a seminar focusing on the roles of occupational therapy and physiotherapy in HIV management.

Evaluation

The students and clinic staff evaluated the experience positively. The interprofessional, peer-learning model helped the students to discern the distinctiveness of their roles as well as the complementary areas of practice in occupational therapy and physiotherapy. The development of a joint assessment process provided effective service delivery and was less stressful for the clients as they had one as opposed to two separate assessments. Students were assertive, advocated for their roles, and accessed other community resources. The following quote from the students' personal interviews following the placement highlights insights gained from the experience.

>> We really had the freedom to kind of create our own assessments, develop intervention plans and we did that together which was very helpful because we were both able to learn from each other and work

> with a client in a very holistic manner. Because not only do we look
> at the physical aspects of it, but looking at spirituality, cultural influences,
> cognitive status and that kind of thing. So I think the partnership we had
> was a very strong aspect for the placement.

When asked if there were any weaknesses or areas requiring attention, the students both indicated that a 5-week placement was insufficient time. Related to this was a disappointment that not all eligible clients took advantage of the assessment or found the opportunity to work with the students to be desirable. The students were also disappointed that some of the staff physicians were unfamiliar with their roles, particularly occupational therapy, and as a result did not always refer appropriate patients. The students realized, however, that a greater length of time would be necessary to build long-term relationships with the clients and clinic staff and market the program effectively.

2. The Transitional Home for Women with Addictions

How It all Started

Many innovative placements start very simply with an expressed need from a community site or a passionate interest from a self-directed student. Jan was a student occupational therapist who submitted an idea to the faculty placement coordinator for a placement in a community, transitional living environment for women in early recovery from addictions to alcohol and drugs. Jan was very interested in this practice area and she was also concerned that this content was not covered in sufficient depth within the curriculum. Additionally there were not many placements offered in the area of addictions. The focus of the transitional home was to provide opportunities to share space with women in early recovery as they work towards maintaining sobriety and work towards recovery. There was no occupational therapist or physiotherapist as part of the staff complement. The program was in need of rehabilitation services and unfortunately did not have the funding to accommodate these services within their existing budget.

The Program Director welcomed the proposal with enthusiasm and support, and played a key role in the success of the placement. She was invaluable in approving the idea, promoting the potential role with her staff, providing a welcoming climate for the student, and ensuring the educational focus of the experience.

Student Perspectives and Outcomes

Jan understood that she was participating in a new and exciting experience. She was carving a role for herself, for the occupational therapy profession, and also representing McMaster University. She realized that she carried responsibility on her shoulders that could pave the way for future links between McMaster University and the site. Jan excelled in the program. It afforded her the opportunity to conduct a needs assessment for the residents, design program plans, and develop a resident resource book. She developed such a positive relationship with the program that she continued to be involved after completing the placement. Through the work that Jan initiated at the transitional home, she established the framework for subsequent student placements, as well as the draft proposal for the development of a funded position for an occupational therapist.

Supervision

Jan realized in the beginning that even though the university and the site supported the proposal, we still had to access a suitable preceptor. Ultimately, two people, the university faculty and a community clinician, supervised Jan. This pairing enabled the faculty to maintain a role in monitoring the experience and liaising with the Program Director. Additionally, the clinician received mentorship from the faculty regarding supervision strategies in a role-emerging placement and was comfortable supervising students in these types of placements in the future at this site.

3. The International Placement: Forging New Roles Abroad

How It Started

Unique opportunities for role-emerging placements exist internationally. Sarah was a student physiotherapist who had a passionate interest in working in an area of a developing country where health human resources and supplies were limited. As this was Sarah's final clinical placement, her goal was to apply physiotherapy practice across the health spectrum from promotion to rehabilitation and reintegration in a rural setting working with a different culture in a developing country. She also wanted to introduce and advocate for the benefits of physiotherapy in the treatment of children with HIV.

Sarah found a preceptor in Kenya through the World Confederation for Physical Therapy who was prepared to supervise her. Aside from physiotherapists employed in the larger hospital settings, her preceptor was the only physiotherapist for the province in which she stayed. His primary focus was to support children needing rehabilitation in a province in Kenya; however, he was not actively involved in the rehabilitation of HIV clients.

This role-emerging placement gave Sarah the freedom she needed to meet her learning needs. She worked closely with her preceptor for the first 10 days of her placement while she learned more about the culture, environment, and health issues in the area. After this she worked independently or was supervised by a nurse who visited HIV clients in their homes. Each night Sarah reviewed her experiences with her preceptor using a case review approach. Her preceptor provided consultation and advice on how to manage her clients.

Opportunities and Challenges

Sarah experienced challenges associated with working in developing countries and in an international context. She had to adjust to the available resources and practice norms of her new environment. For example, neither the clinic where she worked occasionally nor her accommodation had electricity or running water. She often had to travel to remote sites to see HIV-positive clients in their homes where clinical supplies were limited or non-existent.

Differences in teaching and learning styles were notable. One area that presented as a challenge and as an opportunity was how feedback was addressed. Sarah shared her experiences with her preceptor regarding the importance and value of giving and receiving feedback. In doing so, Sarah learned to advocate for a particular teaching/learning approach that was not the norm within this particular international environment. As well, her preceptor learned additional skills that served to enhance his repertoire of clinical teaching skills.

Lessons Learned

As with other international and role-emerging placements, the need for planning many months in advance was evident. Sarah had to be both innovative and sensitive to cultural differences and also to possess knowledge and skills to facilitate the evolution of roles.

Sarah had been asked to provide education to clinicians on HIV rehabilitation. However, she found it was necessary to first describe evidence-based practice so the clinicians could better understand the concepts and rationale for this direction in context to Canadian practice. The clinicians could then subsequently apply these concepts to their own practice.

In role-emerging placements it is also necessary to consider the sustainability of the intervention. It is important not to create a need or expectation only to leave it unmet when the student leaves. To this end, Sarah presented her experiences to other faculty and students on her return to Canada. Her enthusiasm prompted two additional students to complete their final clinical placements in the same location. She developed an orientation package for students who would follow to continue development of this emerging role for physiotherapists. Her goal in doing so was to help shorten the orientation period and to provide some structure to this learning experience. This would lessen the anxiety that future students might have about participating in this placement. Sarah's continuing initiatives are helping to ensure that physiotherapists continue to meet the needs of this population.

Role-emerging placements can provide a unique opportunity for learning both advocacy and leadership skills. Sarah attended a world HIV conference while in Kenya, where Stephen Lewis, United Nations Ambassador for HIV, was speaking. As a fellow Canadian, she took the opportunity to introduce herself and present her plan to seek funding to promote the development of physiotherapy in the prevention and treatment of HIV/AIDS in Kenya. Their relationship continues to this day.

Sarah summarized her experience by stating, "This experience challenged me to be creative and use the knowledge I had obtained in clinical and academic practice to be applied within every different setting. I felt empowered and amazed at my own ability to thrive within this environment."

Etcheverry E (1994) The role of the university faculty in fieldwork. Can J Occup Ther 61:4–43

Farrow S, Gaiptman B, Rudman D (2000) Exploration of a group model in fieldwork education. Can J Occup Ther 67:239–249

Gaiptman B, Forma L (1991) The split placement model for fieldwork placements. Can J Occup Ther 58:85–88

Green S (1996) Traveling via Delphi: a new route to the accreditation of fieldwork educators. Br J Occup Ther 59:506–510

Hamlin RB, MacCrae N, DeBrakeleer B (1995) Will the Opacich fieldwork model work? Am J Occup Ther 49:165–167

Heubner J, Tryssenaar J (1996) Development of an occupational therapy practice perspective in a homeless shelter: a fieldwork experience. Can Assoc Occup Ther 63:24–32

hooks b (1994) Teaching to transgress: education as the practice of freedom. Routledge, New York, NY

hooks b (2003) Teaching community: a pedagogy of hope. Routledge, New York, NY

Hurley L (2000) Funding of clinical education in Ontario university rehabilitation science programs. Council of Ontario Universities, Toronto, ON

Jensen G, Denton B (1991) Teaching physical therapy students to reflect: a suggestion for clinical educators. J Phys Ther Educ 5:33–38

Jung B, Martin A, Graden L, Awrey J (1994) Fieldwork education: a shared supervision model. Can J Occup Ther 61:12–19

Ladyshewsky R (1995) Enhancing service productivity in acute settings using a collaborative clinical education model. Phys Ther 75:504–510

Law M, Baptiste S, Carswell A, McColl M, Polatajko H, Pollock N (1998) The Canadian Occupational Performance Measure (COPM), 3rd edn. CAOT Publications, Ottawa, ON

Maestri A (1996) PT for patients with psychiatric disorders. PT Magazine 4:54–57

Mason J (1998) Fieldwork education: collaborative group learning in community settings. Aust Occup Ther J 45:124–130

Miller BK, Ishler KJ (2001) The rural elderly assessment project: a model for interdisciplinary team training. Occup Ther Health Care 15:3–34

Miller P, Solomon P, Giacomo M, Abelson J (2002) Experiences of novice physiotherapists adapting to their role in acute care hospitals. Physiother Can 57:1–9

Nixon S, Cott C (2000) Shifting perspectives: reconceptualizing HIV disease in a rehabilitation framework. Physiother Can 52:189–197

Perkins J (1996) Reflective journals: suggestions for educators. J Phys Ther Educ 10:8–13

Pontello K, Tryssenaar J (1996) Developing and maintaining emerging role fieldwork sites: a self-directed manual. Partners in Rehab, Thunder Bay, ON

Prigg A, Mackenzie L (2000) Project placements for undergraduate occupational therapy students: design, implementation and evaluation. Occup Ther Int 9:210–236

Sloggett K, Kim N, Cameron D (2003) Private practice: benefits and strategies of providing placements. Can J Occup Ther 70:42–50

Solomon P, Sanford J (1993) Innovative models of student supervision in a home care setting: a pilot project. J Phys Ther Educ 7:49–52

Solomon P, Jung B, Cole B, Beauregard C, Carson E (2003) An innovative clinical education model: developing emerging roles in HIV/AIDS. Poster session presented at the 14th International World Council of Physical Therapy Congress, Barcelona, Spain

Soltys P, Johns S, Sullivan T (1997) A role-emerging fieldwork success story. National 14:5

Strohschein J, Hagler P, May L (2002) Assessing the need for change in clinical education practices. Physiotherapy 82:160–172

Sullivan T, Finlayson M (2000) Role-emerging fieldwork: the University of Manitoba experience. Occup Ther Now 2:13–14

Taylor J, McGlynn-Vittori M, Ellerton C (1997) A conceptual role-shift model: shaping and defining future physical therapy in hospital settings. Physiother Can 49:171–177

Tiberious R, Gaiptman B (1985) The supervisor-student ratio 1:1 versus 1:2. Can J Occup Ther 52:179–183

Tompson M, Proctor JF (1990) Factors affecting a clinician's decision to provide fieldwork education to students. Can J Occup Ther 63:173–182

Tryssenaar J (1994) Interactive journals: an educational strategy to promote reflection. Am J Occup Ther 49:695–702

Van Manen M (2002) The tact of teaching: the meaning of pedagogical thoughtfulness. Althouse, London, ON

Westmorland M, Jung B (1997) Educational partnerships: student and faculty involvement. Br J Ther Rehabil 4:671–675

Wilkins S, Jung B (2002) Establishing research, fieldwork and service partnerships. Phys Occup Ther Geriatr 19:65–78

4

Chapter 5

Evidence-based Practice for the Rehabilitation Sciences

5

Patricia Solomon, Lori Letts

The evidence-based practice (EBP) movement has become very popular within the health professions. The movement started with evidence-based medicine and was led by a group from McMaster University in the early 1990s (Evidence-based Medicine Working Group 1992). It has flourished in the intervening decade. The rehabilitation professions have embraced the movement; textbooks have been written (e.g., Law 2002a), websites have been developed (e.g., Physiotherapy Evidence Database [PEDro], www.otseeker.com), and entire journals have been devoted to the subject (e.g., Physiotherapy Theory and Practice 17, 2001; Canadian Journal of Occupational Therapy 65(3), 1998; 70(5), 2003).

There are several definitions of EBP with one of the most widely quoted coming from Sackett et al. (2000 p. 1) who in this instance refers to evidence-based medicine:

> » Evidence based medicine is the integration of best research evidence with clinical expertise and patient values.

There is increasing recognition that different professions have developed different approaches and have varying definitions of EBP (Dubouloz et al. 1999; Straker 1999). More specific to occupational therapy and physiotherapy, Law (2002b) offers the term evidence-based rehabilitation, which she states is a subset of EBP. She states that four concepts are important to evidence-based rehabilitation: *awareness* of current evidence, *consultation* with the client, *judgment* as to how to apply the recommendations of EBP to a specific client, and *creativity* in applying EBP to specific clients and practice settings. Taylor (2003) notes that even within the rehabilitation professions, occupational therapy and physiotherapy vary in their interpretations. What is clear from reviewing various definitions is that EBP is not a rigidly prescribed approach and requires clinical judgment and acumen to be implemented with individual clients.

Why are EBP skills important for tomorrow's leaders within the rehabilitation professions? As has been noted throughout this book and by many others, the context of today's health care environment is one of information explosion, rapid change, and increased accountability. As a result skills in accurate and efficient information retrieval and critical appraisal of resources to determine the most effective treatment approaches have become essential. However, EBP goes beyond this. For example, an understanding of the principles of outcome measures, their salient psychometric properties, and how to select the correct measure for your purpose is necessary not only for making decisions at the individual client level but also for program evaluation and determination of cost effectiveness (Beattie 2001). Being aware of the properties of diagnostic tests will assist in the selection of the best tests (Stratford 2001). Knowing more about the effectiveness of home modifications to prevent falls may assist occupational therapists in identifying clients most likely to benefit from a prevention program (Cumming et al. 1999). Perhaps the biggest challenge is in going beyond being a "critical consumer" of the literature; that is applying the information to individual patients within the context of a specific practice. We believe that students must be given ample opportunity to practice their EBP decision making in different settings with different populations to best reinforce evidence-based principles and practices.

The intent of this chapter is not to be prescriptive with regards to specific content that should be included in an entry-level rehabilitation science curriculum. When determining curriculum priorities, we feel that it is important, however, for curriculum committees to debate the extent to which professional curricula should prepare students in research methods. The value of requiring research projects of professional students has been questioned (Rothstein 1992). Rothstein (1992) argues that entry-level research projects give students a false sense of the research process, do not contribute to the development of research, and interfere with faculty productivity. A "hands-on" research experience in which students struggle with ethical, methodological, and analytic issues will provide valuable learning. However, the time required to provide this experience has to be debated within the context of ever-competing demands within the curriculum and the need for knowledge and practice of other EBP skills. An independent project may not be feasible in a professional curriculum or may be completed at the expense of developing clinical skills. Group projects may more realistically approximate current research models which are more likely to occur in teams. A recent survey found that over 50 percent of a graduating physiotherapy class participated in a research or program evaluation project in their first three years of practice (Solomon et al. 2004), suggesting that therapists need some fundamental research skills. Does involvement in a small component of an existing faculty project allow students to appreciate the complexities of "doing" research? Is it important to allow professional students an experiential research component to encourage them to proceed to advanced research degrees? Curricular decisions will be influenced by institutional policies and expectations, however, debate on the expected outcomes of graduates with regards to EBP and research expertise is important as the professions grapple with how best to prepare rehabilitation science graduates for current and future health care environments. It may be useful to consider both the skills required to be consumers of evidence and those required to generate evidence (which may include participation in research projects), as well as the most effective teaching methods to promote knowledge transfer to future clinical practice.

Evidence-based practice is dependent on clinicians to incorporate the principles into their clinical decision making. Although the movement is popular in rehabilitation sciences, changes to clinical practice have been slow. Numerous barriers have been identified with a lack of adequate preparation and knowledge being key. More current curricula include EBP content and skills leading to the belief that once there are sufficient numbers of therapists educated in EBP knowledge and skills, EBP will be the "norm". Therefore there are significant expectations for educational programs to prepare graduates who will be well versed in EBP and able to implement changes in the clinical environment. This chapter will discuss some of the challenges to integrating EBP into practice and provide suggestions and examples on how to promote an evidence-based culture within an educational program.

Current Views of the Rehabilitation Professions

In spite of the increasing popularity of EBP in the rehabilitation sciences, barriers to implementation in clinical practice remain. Maintaining a positive attitude toward EBP appears to be difficult with a persistent tendency to rely on "tradition-based" practice following graduation. Connelly et al. (2001) demonstrated that attitudes and perceptions toward research changed positively when they surveyed physiotherapy students prior to and following research methods courses. However, when surveyed one year post-graduation these changes were not maintained. Once in clinical practice the therapists' beliefs about authority of treatment decisions were not sustained and the therapists tended to endorse decisions based on expert opinion rather than research evidence. The reliance on clinical expertise and opinion is widespread. Turner and Whitfield (1999) surveyed physiotherapists in England and Australia to determine their reasons for selection of treatment techniques specifically examining whether "tradition" or research guided their decisions. In both countries the most frequently cited reason for selecting a treatment was that it was "taught in initial training." Journal literature was cited as a reason in 5 percent or less of clinical decisions. Dubouloz et al. (1999), in a qualitative study of eight occupational therapists, found that clinical experience, client input, on the job training, and other colleagues had the greatest influence on clinical decision making. While research was acknowledged as being an important contributor in the decision-making process, it was viewed as secondary to existing methods of carrying out interventions.

Egan and colleagues (2003) conducted an online research project with 49 Canadian occupational therapists, working in isolation from their peers due to time or geographical constraints, to develop practical methods to enhance their use of research findings in practice. The therapists were divided into four working groups based on their areas of practice: institution-based adult rehabilitation, community-based adult rehabilitation, child health, and mental health. Each group connected through asynchronous online conferences with facilitators hired by the project to connect with each group. By the end of the project 20 therapists were still involved. The main result of this study was the production of a seven-step strategy for increasing research use in everyday practice: (1) Determine a practice question, (2) Obtain administrative support, (3) Use reliable sources for information, (4) Apply a theoretical framework to synthesize new information, (5) Use evidence-based methods to critique sources of information, (6) Organize results for clinical decision making, and (7) Share results. Although there were challenges with the use of online technologies, the project resulted in the identification of prerequisites for successful participation and of strategies to optimize online action research, which will be important in future initiatives.

It is important for educators to familiarize students with current views and perceptions on EBP to promote transfer of evidence-based knowledge from the academic to the clinical setting. Students who are aware of the barriers and have discussed and debated potential solutions will be better prepared to act as change agents when they enter clinical practice. The barriers identified are often related to misconceptions about EBP. Many of the misconceptions, originally identified by Sackett et al. (1996), have been portrayed in the occupational therapy and physiotherapy literature; other barriers unique to the rehabilitation professions have also emerged. There is a common belief that there must be one correct way to practice found in the literature, in order for a practitioner to be evidence-based. In a journal editorial, Di Fabio (1999) argues that clinical research is often ignored in the clinical setting because there is insufficient evidence regarding the "right" way to deliver care. He argues that because interpretation of the literature is required to be evidence-based there can be no "absolute truth". Further he claims that EBP cannot be achieved since the practice environment is seldom similar to those described in research settings thus requiring clinicians to make inferences.

However, EBP does not imply that there is one correct way to proceed; rather it recognizes that clinical decisions are based on the integration of evidence, clinicians' expertise, and patient/client preferences. In another editorial, Moore and Petty (2001 p. 196) also express concern that there is a lack of "Grade I RCT studies on which to base [their] practice." They maintain that by relying solely on high levels of evidence therapists may move toward a "recipe book" treatment approach. Their views highlight another misconception that clinical expertise is overlooked in favor of the evidence and that lower levels of evidence are not used in evidence-based decision making. Moseley et al. (2002), in fact, found there was a significant body of knowledge accumulating to guide physiotherapy practice. As of January 2002, there were 2,712 randomized controlled trials (RCTs) and 411 systematic reviews in the PEDro database (Moseley et al. 2002). Law (2002b) contends that the myth that EBP ignores experience and expertise is one of the greatest obstacles to the adoption of EBP. In some instances, the conviction with which clinical experts defend their practice, in spite of a preponderance of negative findings, is alarming (Binkley 2000; Di Fabio 1999).

Yet another misconception encountered, which is particularly salient to rehabilitation practitioners, is that EBP ignores the perceptions of the client and the emphasis is primarily on the practitioner to evaluate the evidence. While concerns related to whether EBP is relevant to individual patients have resonated most strongly in the occupational therapy literature, the argument for the EBP movement to include systematic evaluation of input from clients has also arisen in the physiotherapy literature (Ritchie 1999). EBP has been viewed as being in conflict with the values inherent in client-centered practice (Egan et al. 1999). However, it is clear when reviewing EBP definitions and models of decision making in the rehabilitation sciences that clients' preferences and perspectives are integral to the process (e.g., Canadian Association of Occupational Therapy 1999; Law 2002b).

Another source of confusion in evidence-based rehabilitation is the incorporation of evidence from qualitative research into EBP decision making. The importance of involving the client and including the client in clinical decision making has drawn attention to the value of qualitative methods as sources of evidence to evaluate and integrate into clinical decision making. Qualitative methods, which have roots in the social sciences, have not been historically incorporated into evidence-based medicine, which has roots in the quantitative sciences. Since the EBP model embraced by the rehabilitation professions grew from the evidence-based medicine movement, it is not surprising that there has been little appreciation of the importance of qualitative methods in the early adoption of EBP. Cusick (2001 p. 109) sees this as a problem for professions that are client-centered as "qualitative research provides evidence about the human experience and perception that cannot be accessed any other way." Ritchie (2001) argues that the context in rehabilitation is unique to the individual. She maintains that findings from qualitative studies complement those from quantitative studies and provide important information about the context. As qualitative methods have become more accepted in the health sciences, criteria have been developed to assist in evaluation of the research methods (e.g., Cochrane/Campbell Qualitative Methods Group; Law 2002a).

Another barrier to implementation is the widespread notion that EBP is too time consuming to be practical within a busy clinical practice (Humphris et al. 2000; Huijbregts et al. 2002). There seems to be a lack of appreciation that engaging in EBP does not mean that the best evidence is sought for each and every clinical uncertainty (Herbert et al. 2001). Judicious use of evidence means that the clinician prioritizes important clinical questions. Herbert et al. (2001 p. 204) state "much of clinical practice is far from optimally effective and that potentially even modest amounts of time spent in the judicious application of evidence to clinical decision making could substantially improve clinical outcomes". Sackett et al. (2000) outline a number of strategies to integrate EBP in hospital and community settings that are salient to all health care practitioners and educators. These include a model for a journal club, group sessions, or "academic half days" and the use of critically appraised topics (CATs) which are one-page summaries outlining a clinical question, appraising the literature, and presenting a clinical "bottom line" based on the evidence.

There seems to be another belief that EBP refers primarily to questions related to interventions and effectiveness and that only the RCT is an acceptable level of evidence. For example, Bithell (2000) states that EBP bases its judgments on a hierarchy of methodologies best suited to the clinical testing of the efficacy of drugs and argues against using the RCT as "best evidence" in rehabilitation sciences. Moore claims that there is a danger that clinicians "may pay no heed to other evidence, albeit at a lower level in the hierarchy" (Moore and Petty 2001 p. 196). Not only is EBP more than looking at effectiveness studies, a lack of RCTs does not imply that no treatment be administered. Sackett et al. (1996 p. 72) state that if there is no RCT one must follow "the trail to the next best external evidence." It is also important to consider the best level of evidence available for the type of question asked. For example, if a question is related to clients' experiences with cognitive–behavioral interventions, qualitative research may be the best evidence to answer the question.

In summary, there are a number of misconceptions and related barriers to implementation that are prevalent within the rehabilitation science professions. Students need to be prepared, not only with the knowledge and skills to search, evaluate and integrate EBP into clinical decision making but also with the skills to confront barriers, educate others, and implement changes in professional practice.

Strategies for Developing an Evidence-based Culture

The barriers to EBP can make it difficult for students to translate knowledge and skills from the academic to the clinical setting. If EBP is not valued and reinforced in clinical practice, students and new graduates may revert to practice based solely on clinical expertise. In our view, it is important to develop an evidence-based culture that permeates through all components of a curriculum in order for students to value and support this as an essential element of practice. Ideally, integration in the curriculum is both horizontal and vertical. Horizontal integration ensures that the content area is streamed across all semesters of study. Vertical integration ensures that EBP is an element of all courses within a semester of study, including theoretical, practical, and clinical education courses. Table 5.1 provides an overview of horizontal and vertical integration of EBP as organized in the Occupational Therapy Program at McMaster University. Faculty chose to describe EBP in two parts: consuming and generating evidence. In the first two terms of study, emphasis is on developing skills in consuming evidence (with application of evidence in practice receiving more attention at the end of year 1). Participation and learning about generating evidence begins in the third term and continues throughout the program. Assignments and expectations build in each area throughout the six terms of study. The following sections demonstrate how EBP principles can be integrated into a variety of learning contexts.

Problem-based Learning

The problem-based learning (PBL) model of curriculum design can assist in promoting and reinforcing an evidence-based culture. Although there are many variations of PBL (Barrows 1986), typically the process focuses on the following steps: (1) students are presented with a health care problem which forms the basis for initial discussion and problem solving, (2) through the discussion students generate questions for self-study that will assist them in understanding issues that arise in the problem, (3) students search for resources to assist in understanding questions, and engage in self-directed study, (4) students synthesize and apply information to the health care problem, and (5) the process is evaluated (Barrows and Tamblyn 1980). The health care problems are carefully designed to elicit learning related to many content areas including basic, clinical, and psychosocial sciences as well as EBP. Although not universal, most often PBL occurs in a small group tutorial setting with the assistance of a faculty tutor who assumes the role of facilitator of information rather than of knowledge expert. Examination of components of this process will illustrate how EBP can be reinforced through the PBL approach.

Problem Design

The problem can be designed to integrate and highlight specific EBP objectives. While the primary objective of the problem may be related to increasing the understanding of, for example, pathophysiology of stroke and various treatment approaches, cues in the problem can lead to learning objectives that reinforce EBP. The problem scenario could include an anxious relative who asks the question of whether the client will be able to walk again thus prompting the students to develop a learning issue related to natural history of stroke and prognosis. Findings from an assessment tool which is unfamiliar to the students can steer them to examine the measurement properties of the tool. Or a specific treatment approach may lead to the question of effectiveness of the treatment. Alternatively, the problem may be designed with EBP objectives as the primary focus. For example, an assignment in the first term of the occupational therapy program focuses on having pairs of students search the recent occupational therapy literature for evidence that contributes directly to one of two case scenarios, specifically designed to raise a number of questions related to evidence supporting occupational therapy practice. Students search, critically appraise the article, and consider its application to the scenario. They are evaluated on a one-page summary of the information as well as on the presentation of the evidence and its application within the context of the tutorial session.

Formulating Questions for Self-study

An important EBP skill is the ability to articulate a clear, searchable study question. Richardson et al. (1995) see this as a fundamental skill for an evidence-based practitioner. They state that a well-articulated question has four components: (1) the patient or problem being addressed, (2) the intervention or exposure being considered, (3) the comparison intervention or exposure, and (4) the clinical outcome of interest. Although this format works only for questions related to intervention effectiveness, and not all EBP questions are related to interventions, the model of asking clear and specific questions is an important one for students to apply. Learning to ask good quality questions is a critical element in both the PBL and EBP processes. Students quickly learn that it is difficult to search and obtain relevant information if the question is vague or non-specific. Asking "How do you manage elbow pain?" will be much more difficult to search and answer than "Is ultrasound effective in the treatment of lateral epicondylitis?" Similarly, it is easier to find evidence to answer the question "Which functional assessment instrument(s) designed to evaluate cognition are most appropriate for use with clients with acquired brain injury in their homes? community setting?" than "Which cognitive assessments are most appropriate for use in the community?"

5

Table 5.1. Evidence-based practice content across the occupational therapy curriculum. (*PBT* Problem-based tutorial, *PREP* professional roles and experiential practicum, *EBP* evidence-based practice, *CAA* critical appraisal assignment, *EBAA* evidence-based appraisal of assessment, *EBAI* evidence-based appraisal of intervention)

	Term 1 (PBT)	Term 2 (PBT Practicum)	Term 3 (PBT Practicum)	Term 4 (PBT Practicum)	Term 5 (PBT)	Term 6 (PBT Practicum)
Consuming evidence Develop questions	Library sessions PREP session briefly			EBP seminar – dilemmas EBP large group session		
Search evidence	Library intro PBT critical appraisal assignment	PREP EBAA Inquiry scholarly paper and class presentation	PREP EBAI	EBP seminar – dilemmas	EBP large group session on advanced knowledge to appraise clinical practice guidelines	
Critical appraisal	PREP CAA PBT CAA	PREP EBAA Inquiry scholarly paper and class presentation	PREP EBAI Inquiry evidence-based decision-making session	EBP seminar – dilemmas	EBP group critical appraisal presentation	
Summarize evidence	PREP CAA PBT CAA	PREP EBAA Inquiry scholarly paper and class presentation	PREP EBAI Inquiry evidence-based decision-making session	EBP seminar – dilemmas	EBP large group session re outcomes EBP group critical appraisal presentation	
Integrate and apply to practice	Informal in PBT Info session with tutors and students	PREP EBAA	PREP EBAI Inquiry evidence-based decision-making session PREP modified essay question examination (some students)	EBP seminar – dilemmas	EBP group critical appraisal presentation EBP large group session re outcomes	EBP reflective paper on applying evidence in practice EBP large group session on becoming an evidence-based practitioner

Generating evidence Formulate question			Inquiry mini-qualitative research assignment	EBP projects EBP large group session	EBP projects/ practicum	EBP projects EBP research proposal assignment
Design research – quantitative and qualitative			Inquiry mini-qualitative research assignment	EBP projects EBP large group sessions	EBP projects/ practicum EBP session re harm, prognosis, tests	EBP research proposal assignment EBP projects
Program evaluation				EBP projects (some students) Web-based course and assignments	EBP projects/ practicum (some students)	EBP projects (some students) Program proposal paper
Ethics review				EBP projects EBP large group session	EBP projects/ practicum	
Data collection and analysis			Inquiry mini-qualitative research assignment	EBP projects (some students)	EBP projects/ practicum (some students) EBP large group statistics and analysis sessions	EBP projects (some students)
Integrate evidence in practice			Inquiry mini-qualitative research assignment		EBP seminar groups on applica-tion of evidence to practice	EBP seminar groups on application of evidence to practice
Disseminate					EBP large group seminar	EBP project presentations and reports

5

Searching for Resources

Being able to efficiently access resources to address learning questions is also a fundamental skill of the evidence-based practitioner. While students access a variety of written and people resources, a component of the tutorial process typically includes performing a literature search to assist in addressing the questions they have formulated for self-study. Students develop literature searching skills and become familiar with the strengths and weaknesses of the various databases.

Synthesis and Application to the Patient Problem

Through role modeling and appropriate questioning the faculty tutor can reinforce many evidence-based elements. For example, the tutor can ask questions related to how the student's literature search led to a specific article, the level of evidence to support a recommended treatment intervention, or whether there is any research to support the reliability and validity of a specific assessment tool.

Evaluation

Also typical in the PBL process is the use of dedicated time to evaluate group and individual performance at the end of each tutorial. Evaluation criteria may include objectives specific to EBP to further reinforce its importance to the clinical decision-making process. The tutor and the students are actively engaged in the evaluation and may discuss the quality of the learning questions generated for self-study, the relative success of the search strategies used to seek information, the quality of the information retrieved, the accuracy of the critical appraisal and its application to scenarios discussed, and areas where further research is required.

It is important to note that the problems integrate many elements of physiotherapy or occupational therapy practice and EBP is one of many content areas that will be reinforced to a greater or lesser extent dependent on concurrent curricular goals. It is through consistent reinforcement and expectations that students learn to ask high-level searchable questions, conduct efficient searches, evaluate the literature, and integrate the findings in the clinical decision making related to the problem. Table 5.2 summarizes how various aspects of EBP can be promoted through the PBL process.

Tutors play a significant role in ensuring the tutorial groups search, appraise, and apply evidence. Therefore, it is essential that tutors are supported in developing and enhancing their own knowledge and skill in EBP. This is especially important early in the curriculum, when students are learning about the processes of PBL and expectations are clearly laid out for future terms. If tutors are representatives from the clinical community, the expectations of students need to be made clear to them and to the students. Regular meetings with tutors can clarify expectations and provide opportunities for the tutors to develop facilitation and evaluation skills to best support the students. Vignettes can be used to illustrate how tutors can challenge tutorial groups to apply EBP in PBL.

Table 5.2. Using problem-based learning (PBL) to promote development of evidence-based practice (EBP) skills

Step in PBL	How EBP promoted
1. Discussion of health care problem	Group discussion highlights and reinforces select EBP principles
2. Generation of questions for self-study	Students learn to develop clear, researchable questions
3. a) Search for resources b) Self-directed study	Students develop literature searching skills
4. a) Synthesize information b) Apply to health care problem	Direct application of EBP skills to health care problem
5. Evaluation	Feedback on skills, reinforcement of EBP principles

Clinical Skills Courses

As previously mentioned, to promote an evidence-based culture, it is important that students view EBP as an expectation for all courses, not just courses related to research or theoretical aspects of practice. In the physiotherapy program the clinical skills courses are designed to complement and reinforce content introduced in the small group tutorial setting. A recurring theme in the course is the application of clinical measurement principles. A clinical skill is divided into three components: the technical skill, obtaining the result, and interpreting the meaning of the result for a specific patient. For example, if one measures knee joint range of motion, the technical skill is the correct application of the goniometer, obtaining the result combines the measurement concept of averaging to reduce error and reading the goniometer correctly, and applying the result to a specific patient is the ability to interpret the same finding differently on different clients (e.g., 112 degrees of knee flexion on a 15-year-old with a postoperative anterior cruciate ligament repair compared to a 74-year-old postoperative patient with a total knee replacement).

Table 5.3 provides an example of how content in a PBL tutorial course and a clinical skills course can be integrated vertically in a typical week of study. This approach works successfully in the physiotherapy program, since students work through specific problems each week so the learning across courses is complementary. In this example, the description of the health care problem includes some client data related to clinical findings on examination. As this is early in the curriculum, some fundamental learning issues are generated. The clinical skills course focuses on the principles of application of goniometry i.e., the "skills" component. In addition, relevant concepts of principles of measurement are introduced in context to highlight clinical relevancy. After students engage in self-directed study they have an additional tutorial session where content related to the learning issues is discussed, debated, and applied to the client in the health care problem. Further information is provided and students generate additional learning issues.

In the occupational therapy program, clinical skills are taught through the Professional Roles and Experiential Practicum (PREP) courses, which also include the clinical education component of the program. In the first term of the program, the PREP

Table 5.3. Example of vertical integration of evidence-based practice in the curriculum

Day 1	PROBLEM-BASED TUTORIAL COURSE
	FIRST TUTORIAL
	
	Range of motion (ROM) data provided in the health care problem
	Student learning questions:
	    How do you measure ROM?
	    Are there normative values?
	    How confident can you be in your measures?
	    (Introduce concept of reliability)

Day 2	CLINICAL SKILLS COURSE
	
	Focus on goniometry and reliability
	    Six students measure active ROM in the same six students
	    Examine concepts – standard error of the measurement,
	    minimal detectable change

Day 3	SELF-DIRECTED STUDY
Day 4	PROBLEM-BASED TUTORIAL COURSE SECOND TUTORIAL Additional patient data includes reassessment of ROM Students use literature to determine whether minimal detectable change has reoccurred Apply to patient problem in context of other findings

course provides educational sessions addressing the skills associated with critical appraisal. There is an assignment that involves pairs of students critically reviewing one quantitative and one qualitative research article and drafting a memo integrating and applying the results in a practice setting. EBP principles are integrated horizontally throughout the PREP courses. For example, the second term, which has a focus on assessment across the lifespan, includes an assignment to critically appraise an assessment that is commonly used in occupational therapy practice. Term 3 has a similar assignment for students to critically appraise an occupational therapy intervention. In terms 2 and 3, students prepare handouts which are posted and made available to their peers, so that students complete each term with a package of current critical reviews of assessments and interventions. Throughout all six terms of study, students, faculty, and guest speakers are encouraged to apply the best evidence available when considering the skills that are being taught and learned.

Clinical Education

Clinical education presents unique challenges to reinforcing EBP. As Richardson (1999) suggests there is often a sense that academic and clinical cultures are very different. This can require students to "unlearn" and "relearn" knowledge in the clinical setting and can disrupt continuity in the clinical setting. Clinical supervisors who may have graduated prior to inclusion of EBP into professional curricula may not role model behaviors or value the questioning attitude that the student portrays. In earlier attempts to promote EBP in clinical education, students were provided with learning objectives related to critical appraisal to complete during their clinical education placements (Solomon and Stratford 1992). The model proved to be difficult for some

Table 5.4. Example of evidence-based practice assignment in clinical education

For this placement two evidence-based summary assignments should be completed, one related to an assessment question and one related to a treatment question. For each question:

1. Identify a patient or client from your clinical practice.

2. Describe the chief complaint or presenting problem.

3. State the clinical question that is a concern with this patient and that you are trying to address.

4. Identify an article that best informs your clinical decision making related to the clinical question stated in 3.

5. Summarize the article's strengths and weaknesses.

6. State its value to the clinical decision-making process and how you incorporated the findings into your decision-making process of the specific patient/client. Consider the role of your clinical knowledge/expertise and the patient's values and preferences as part of your clinical decision making.

Include your articles with the assignments. The summary should be a maximum of two pages in length. Students are required to present their evidence-based summary at their clinical placement site. This will allow clinicians and other students to benefit from the student's experience.

clinical supervisors who felt they did not have the expertise to evaluate students. Reflecting the practice at the time, the emphasis was on critical appraisal of the literature. Clinical assignments presently reflect more current definitions of EBP. In each clinical setting students are required to complete a brief assignment related to a specific patient and reflect on the patient values and their clinical expertise, in addition to the literature, when making their clinical decisions (Table 5.4). A critical component of the assignment is to encourage dialogue between the student and the clinical supervisor. Through requiring the student to share the assignment with the clinical supervisor and others we hope to encourage dialogue and debate, demystify EBP, and contribute to the knowledge of the clinicians.

Specific Evidence-based Practice Courses

While we feel that it is vital to integrate EBP principles into all components of the curricula to create an evidence-based culture, we have also found value in having some courses that focus exclusively on EBP and research. In the occupational therapy program, for example, the second year of the program includes three full courses that run across three terms of study. As much as possible, these are integrated horizontally with the content of the other large group inquiry, problem-based tutorial, and PREP courses previously mentioned. One of these courses is a large group seminar that focuses on providing students with more in-depth knowledge needed to consume and generate evidence. Sessions include topics such as designing research questions, research ethics, designing quantitative and qualitative studies, and statistical analyses. Learning activities in the course include a web-based component with accompanying assignments related to designing a program evaluation, development of a research proposal using the format and criteria of the Canadian Occupational Therapy Foundation (which is often a first funder for many clinicians interested in research), and working in groups to critically appraise the literature specifically related to a clinical scenario.

5

Table 5.5. Sample practice dilemmas for evidence-based practice small group seminar course

Sample dilemma #1:

Occupational therapists at the City of Hamilton frequently work with sanitation workers who lift hundreds of pounds of garbage into garbage trucks every day. There is some discussion about whether employees are being asked to lift too much (or not enough) in a day and whether these employees are at increased risk for certain types of injury/impairment because of the work they do.

Question: How much repetitive lifting can an employee tolerate (male or female) before he/she significantly increases his/her risk of musculoskeletal injury/impairment (i.e., low back strain, rotator cuff tear, osteoarthritis, etc.)? (Maximum weight of each garbage bag is supposed to be 50 lbs.)

Sample dilemma #2:

Occupational therapists at St Joseph's Hospital in Hamilton spend three to four hours doing home assessments with clients preparing for discharge from rehabilitation units. This often means that there are other patients not being seen by occupational therapists during home visits. Can we justify the time spent away from these patients? Can we establish a protocol for who we should be doing home visits with (i.e., are there some individuals that require them and others who don't)? How will we determine who needs one?

A second course is a small group seminar format, which uses clinical dilemmas as a starting off point. Although these are often similar to scenarios used in the PBL courses, they differ in that the perspective is from the viewpoint of the therapist rather than one specific client. Table 5.5 includes two sample dilemmas. These dilemmas are generated by community clinicians who are invited to submit them to the course coordinator. When students select a dilemma, the clinician is contacted for further information and invited to attend the seminar group when the student will present and discuss the findings. Clinicians also receive a copy of the students' four-page summary of evidence. Faculty facilitators evaluate students on their re-formulation of the question into a searchable format, their search strategies, critical appraisal of the evidence, and application of the evidence to the scenario. The format of this course has been a successful way to demonstrate to students the types of "real" questions that come from clinicians, and to support clinicians by sharing the results with them. It serves to reach out from the academic into the clinical realm to share the evidence-based culture. The final EBP course in the occupational therapy program is the evidence-based project course. Students, alone or in groups of two or three, work with a faculty or community supervisor to participate in a research project. A practicum is devoted to five weeks of full-time work on the projects; additional hours throughout the academic portions of year 2 are also dedicated to this course. Although debate may continue about the value of participating in research, the projects range from formulating questions, collecting data, developing program evaluation, and evaluating outcome measures – initiatives in which occupational therapists in practice commonly participate.

Conclusion

Evidence-based practice is as much to do with developing a questioning and open attitude as it is with developing specific knowledge and skills. A multifaceted approach which streams EBP both horizontally and vertically in the curriculum reinforces the importance of EBP in all components of practice. A consistent message from all faculty reinforces the culture of EBP.

The authors wish to acknowledge Professor Paul Stratford, Professor Mary Tremblay, Shy Amlani, and Melissa Jamieson for contributing to the curricular materials referred to in this chapter.

References

Barrows H (1986) A taxonomy of problem based learning methods. Med Educ 20:481–486
Barrows H, Tamblyn R (1980) Problem-based learning. Springer, Berlin Heidelberg New York
Beattie P (2001) Measurement of health outcomes in the clinical setting: applications to physiotherapy. Physiother Theory Pract 17:173–175
Binkley J (2000) Letter to the editor. J Orthop Sports Phys Ther 30:98–99
Bithell C (2000) Evidence based physiotherapy. Physiotherapy 86:58–60
Canadian Association of Occupational Therapy (1999) Joint position statement on evidence based occupational therapy. Can J Occup Ther 66:267–269
Connolly B, Lupinnaci N, Bush A (2001) Changes in attitudes and perceptions about research in physical therapy among professional physical therapy students and new graduates. Phys Ther 81:1127–1134
Cumming RG, Thomas M, Szonyi G, Salkeld G, O'Neill E, Westbury C, Frampton G (1999) Home visits by an occupational therapist for assessment and modification of environmental hazards: a randomized trial of falls prevention. J Am Geriatr Soc 47:1397–1402
Cusick A (2001) Australian occupational therapy, evidence based practice and the 21st century. Aust J Occup Ther 48:102–117
Di Fabio R (1999) Myth of evidence based practice. J Orthop Sports Phys Ther 29:632–634
Dubouloz CJ, Egan M, Vallerand J, von Zweck C (1999) Occupational therapists' perceptions of evidence based practice. Am J Occup Ther 53:445–453
Egan M, Dubouloz CJ, von Zweck C, Vllerand J (1999) The client centered evidence based practice of occupational therapy. Can J Occup Ther 63:136–143
Egan M, Duboulox CJ, Rappolt S, Polatajko H, von Zweck C, Graham I (2003) Enhancing research use through an on-line action research project: final report. University of Ottawa School of Rehabilitation Sciences, Ottawa, ON
Evidence-based Medicine Working Group (1992) Evidence-based medicine: a new approach to teaching the practice of medicine. JAMA 268:2420–2425
Herbert R, Sherrington C, Maher C, Mosley A (2001) Evidence-based practice: imperfect but necessary. Physiother Theory Pract 17:201–211
Huijbregts M, Myers A, Kay T, Gavin T (2002) Systematic outcome measurement in clinical practice: challenges experienced by physiotherapists. Physiother Can 54:25–31
Humphris D, Littlejohns P, Victor C, O'Halloran P, Peacock J (2000) Implementing evidence based practice: factors that influence the use of research evidence by occupational therapists. Br J Occup Ther 63:516–522
Law M (2002a) Evidence-based rehabilitation: a guide to practice. Slack, Thorofare, NJ
Law M (2002b) Introduction to evidence-based practice. In: Law M (ed) Evidence-based rehabilitation: a guide to practice. Slack, Thorofare, NJ
Moore A, Petty N (2001) Evidence based practice: getting a grip and finding the balance. Man Ther 6:195–196
Moseley A, Herbert R, Sherrington C, Maher C (2002) Evidence for physiotherapy practice: a survey of the physiotherapy evidence database (PEDro). Aust J Physiother 48:43–49
Richardson B (1999) Professional development 2. Professional knowledge and situated learning in the workplace. Physiotherapy 85:467–474
Richardson W, Wilson M, Nishikawa J, Hayward R (1995) The well built clinical question: a key to evidence based decisions. ACP J Club 123:A12–A13
Ritchie J (1999) Using qualitative research to enhance the evidence-based practice of health care providers. Aust J Physiother 45:251–256
Ritchie J (2001) Case series research: a case for qualitative method in assembling the evidence. Physiother Theory Pract 17:127–135
Rothstein J (1992) Living without student research projects. Phys Ther 72:332–333

Sackett D, Rosenberg W, Muir Gray J, Haynes B, Richardson W (1996) Evidence based medicine: what it is and what it isn't. BMJ 312:71–72

Sackett D, Straus S, Richardson W, Rosenberg W, Haynes B (2000) Evidence-based medicine: how to practice and teach EBM, 2nd edn. Churchill Livingstone, New York, NY

Solomon P, Stratford P (1992) Promoting critical appraisal of research literature in the undergraduate. J Phys Ther Educ 6:19–21

Solomon P, Ohman A, Miller P (2004) A follow-up study on career choice and professional socialization in physiotherapists. Physiother Can 56:102–110

Straker L (1999) A hierarchy of evidence for informing physiotherapy practice. Aust J Physiother 45:231–233

Stratford P (2001) Applying the results from diagnostic accuracy studies to enhance clinical decision making. Physiother Theory Pract 17:153–160

Taylor M (2003) Evidence-based practice: informing practice and critically evaluating related research. In: Brown G, Esdaile S, Ryan S (eds) Becoming an advanced health care practitioner. Butterworth Heinemann, London

Turner P, Whitfield T (1999) Physiotherapists' reasons for selection of treatment techniques: a cross national survey. Physiother Theory Pract 15:235–246

Chapter 6

Ethics

6

E. Lynne Geddes, Margaret Brockett

Contents

6

While ethics and ethical issues have been discussed in the rehabilitation literature since the 1970s, there was a significant increase in the number of publications on these topics during the 1990s (Swisher 2002). Not surprisingly, this corresponded with changes in the role of rehabilitation professionals, and in the health care environment, that have resulted in an increase in the complexity and frequency of ethical decision making by occupational therapists and physiotherapists.

The role of rehabilitation professionals has evolved, shifting from "allied health professionals" under the direction of physicians to increasingly autonomous practitioners with independence in and accountability for making clinical decisions (Swisher 2002). Occupational therapists and physiotherapists in Ontario, Canada were recognized as primary health care practitioners with the enactment of the Regulated Health Professions Act, the Occupational Therapy Act, and the Physiotherapy Act in 1991 (e-Laws: Ontario Statutes and Regulations 2004). This led to the creation of self-regulatory colleges with Standards of Practice and Codes of Ethics to which members must comply. Increased autonomy, however, leads to increased complexity of ethical dilemmas encountered in contemporary clinical practice (Swisher 2002). "Ethical decision making and moral virtue are dimensions of clinical expertise rather than separate steps in the process of providing physical therapy" (Swisher 2002 p. 693).

The relationship between patients and practitioners has also changed. Easier access to health care knowledge through advances in information technology has meant that patients are no longer outsiders to the health care system (Kelley 2002). They are able to be active participants in their care, which is quite different from the paternalistic model in which the patient defers to the practitioner's recommendations. This is reflected in changes in terminology from "patient" to "client" to "consumer." Furthermore, patients must consent to the collection, use, and disclosure of their information, and have the right to access their health records and to correct erroneous personal information (Privacy Commissioner of Canada 2004). Recognition of the patient's greater involvement in his/her care has led to increased awareness that the patient may have different values and perspectives from those of the health care practitioner.

While health practitioners have more autonomy, and patients may be more knowledgeable participants, there has also been an increase in team decision making (Kelley 2002), with members seeking to reach consensus before proceeding with a decision (Barnitt 1998). However, each team member brings their own personal and professional cultures and values, particular clinical and ethical reasoning styles, and different professional obligations to the table. Decisions are also influenced by the expectations of the payer of the services and the type of funding model for health care.

Practice has also been influenced by the additional demands that have been placed upon the health care system by advances in scientific knowledge, by the variety and efficacy of medical technologies, by demographic shifts in the population emphasizing care in certain age groups, and by increased life expectancy at both ends of the lifespan. Increased costs and budget restraints have led to wait lists and rationing of limited resources.

Ethics Education in Professional Programs

As a result of these developments, educational programs have recognized the importance of, and need for, ethics education. "New demands for this type of curriculum content come from professional bodies, changing practice in health care, and, in particular, the anxieties that students bring to their [instructors] after clinical or field-work experience" (Barnitt 1993 p. 406).

In 1991, Finley and Goldstein reported on a survey of entry-level physiotherapy education programs in the United States. Of the respondents, over 95 percent included ethical and legal instruction related to physiotherapy in their curricula, with the primary foci being licensing, American Physical Therapy Association Code of Ethics, American Physical Therapy Association Guide of Professional Conduct, documentation, informed consent, and patient rights. Seventy-five percent of the programs had up to 20 hours of instruction, with lecture and large group discussion being the most common methods of presentation. These authors recommended that educators "consider incorporating a broad-based approach to the study of ethical theories and moral decision making into their curricular content" (Finley and Goldstein 1991 p. 63).

Barnitt (1993) conducted a survey of ethics education in occupational therapy and physiotherapy programs within the United Kingdom. Ethics education was included in 16 of the 19 occupational therapy programs and in 18 of the 22 physiotherapy programs who responded, with a range of 1–21 hours of study. The most frequent themes for the content were ethics related to research, professional issues, and clinical experience.

Brockett (1996) and Geddes (1998) replicated Barnitt's (1993) survey with occupational therapy and physiotherapy programs in Canada. All respondents included teaching about ethics in their curricula and all provided students with Codes of Ethics. The hours of instruction ranged from 2 to 20 hours. Respondents felt that ethics ideally should be integrated across the curriculum and 7 of the 10 physiotherapy programs were in the process of implementing curricular changes.

The surveys by Barnitt (1993), Brockett (1996), and Geddes (1998) found that while occupational therapy and physiotherapy programs provided ethics education, the issue of moral reasoning was much less clear. Moral reasoning was defined as "the philosophical inquiry about norms and values, about ideas of right and wrong, good or bad, what should or should not be done, what ought to be done, how you make moral decisions in your professional work". Only three programs answered this section in Barnitt's (1993) study because most of the respondents viewed moral reasoning as synonymous with ethics teaching. While the occupational therapy and physiotherapy programs in Canada felt that moral reasoning should be part of the curricula, Brockett (1996) concluded that occupational therapy programs focused on standards, rules, and regulations with little emphasis on moral theory and moral reasoning, and Geddes (1998) found that the majority of physiotherapy programs did not include moral reasoning in their curricula.

While more traditional formats, such as lectures, have been the main means of providing ethics education, evidence supports the use of small group, case-based learning that is clinically relevant and that promotes group discussion and ethical decision making (Krawczyk 1997; ten Have 1995). Integration of ethics content throughout the curriculum in both academic and clinical settings is advocated (Barnitt 1993; Brockett 1996; Finley and Goldstein 1991; Geddes 1998).

Incorporating Ethics into Physiotherapy and Occupational Therapy Curricula

The Occupational Therapy and Physiotherapy Programs at McMaster University, Hamilton, Ontario are built upon the pedagogical foundation of problem-based learning that is based on the premise that learning is enhanced by: "stimulation of prior knowledge, learning in context to enhance retention, and elaboration of knowledge through discussion" (Saarinen-Rahiika and Binkley 1998 p. 196).

In contrast to traditional educational models that are built around subject-driven courses, problem-based learning provides an integrated curriculum that is driven by the content of the health care problems included in each term of study. There is substantial interdependence within and between terms and among faculty (Solomon and Geddes 2001), and even a small change in the content of a problem may alter the learning that students identify and pursue (Solomon et al. 1992). Different streams of content (such as ethics) are woven across the curriculum within the health care problems. Problem-based learning has been shown to be more effective than traditional course-based models for enhancing students' knowledge of ethics and their skills in moral reasoning and ethical decision making (Goldie et al. 2001).

Through the use of health care problems in the small group setting, selective use of large group classes, and integration of the academic and clinical settings, the Occupational Therapy and Physiotherapy Programs at McMaster University embarked on the development, implementation, and evaluation of ethics content and moral reasoning. The process began in the early to mid 1990s and continues to undergo review and revision. The programs approach the development of ethics streams across their curriculum differently based on three factors:

- Student choice of health care problems. Within the Physiotherapy Program problems are introduced in a more prescribed manner, whereas students in the Occupational Therapy Program choose from a wide selection of problems.

- Ethical reasoning style. Occupational therapists have been shown to prefer a narrative ethical reasoning style to the diagnostic and procedural method of their physiotherapy colleagues (Barnitt and Partridge 1997).

- Personality types using the Myers-Briggs Type Indicator. Physiotherapy students are more likely to be "judgers", preferring structure and organization. The evidence for occupational therapy students is equivocal but may lean toward them being "perceivers," taking a more flexible and spontaneous approach (Hardigan and Cohen 1998; Lysak et al. 2001).

Ethics Education in the Physiotherapy Program

Given the interconnectedness of a problem-based learning curriculum and the potential impact of even small changes in a health care problem, the Physiotherapy Program recognized the need to examine the entire curriculum and to seek faculty consensus when incorporating ethics content. Beginning in 1994, the Program applied a systematic process for implementing the ethics stream within the curriculum. This process has been well described (Geddes et al. 1998, 1999; Solomon and Geddes 2001) and is provided in graphic form in Fig. 6.1.

Evidence in the literature, research conducted by faculty at McMaster University, and the experience of clinicians were all key in identifying the need to address ethics within the curriculum. In order to identify what ethics content to include in the curriculum, a consensus exercise was conducted with faculty, current students, and local clinicians. Faculty and students completed a survey and participated in focus groups.

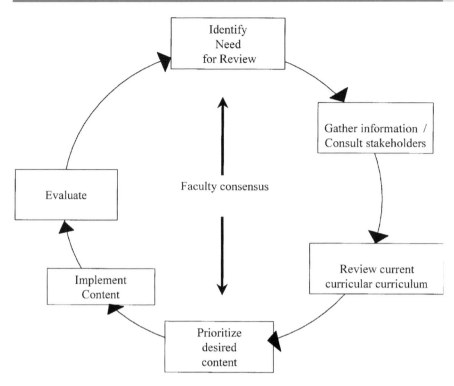

Fig. 6.1. Model of process for ethics content review in the Physiotherapy Program. Reprinted with permission from Solomon P, Geddes EL (2001) A systematic process for content review in a problem-based learning curriculum. Med Teach 23:556–560. http://www.tandf.co.uk/journals

Clinicians participated through mail-in of the survey. Quantitative and qualitative analysis of the consensus exercise resulted in the identification of key ethical issues viewed as important to physiotherapy practice.

The next step consisted of a review of the ethics content in the problems that formed the basis of the physiotherapy curriculum. Two external experts in health care ethics education rated the extent to which ethical issues were included in the problems and the ease with which a novice learner could identify the ethical issue. The evaluators used the list of issues generated from the consensus exercise and added other issues that were repeatedly found in the problems but not explicitly stated through the consensus. The result was the identification of twelve ethical issues for physiotherapy practice (Table 6.1) and the rating of these issues within each health care problem. A sample of the rating key and the grid is provided in Fig. 6.2 (Solomon and Geddes 2001). At the conclusion of this step in the process, faculty within the program with intimate knowledge of the problems cross-validated the results.

A second consensus exercise was held with core faculty with the purpose of determining the desired depth of learning for each of the ethical issues in the curriculum and to stream the ethical issues throughout the program of study. Rating was based on a taxonomy for education objectives for the cognitive domain, with superficial depth being knowledge and/or comprehension of the ethical issue, moderate depth being application, and greater depth being analysis and/or synthesis (Gronlund 1985).

ETHICAL ISSUES	HEALTH CARE - PROBLEMS UNIT 1					UNIT II				UNIT III			
	Problem 1	Problem 2	Problem 3	Problem 4	Problem 5	Problem 1	Problem 2	Problem 3	Problem 4	Problem 1	Problem 2	Problem 3	Problem 4
1. Informed Consent	3/2	3/2	3/2	4/2	2/1		3/2	3/2	3/2	3/2	3/3	4/3	4/3
2. Truth Telling	4/3	4/2	5/3	3/2	5/3	3/2	2/1	4/4	4/3	5/4	4/4	4/3	3/2
3. Privacy / Confidentiality			5/4			3/2	3/1	2/1		3/2	4/2	1/1	1/1
4. Quality of Life	5/5	4/3	4/3	5/4	5/3	3/1	3/2	5/4	4/3	4/3	5/4	3/2	4/3
5. Allocation of Scarce Resources	3/2	3/1	1/1			1/1	3/2		2/1	3/2	2/2	3/2	1/1

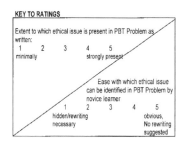

KEY TO RATINGS

Extent to which ethical issue is present in PBT Problem as written:
1   2   3   4   5
minimally   strongly present

Ease with which ethical issue can be identified in PBT Problem by novice learner
1   2   3   4   5
hidden/rewriting necessary   obvious, No rewriting suggested

Fig. 6.2. Grid to evaluate ethics content in the health care problems of the Physiotherapy Program (partial example). Reprinted with permission from Solomon P, Geddes EL (2001) A systematic process for content review in a problem-based learning curriculum. Med Teach 23: 556–560. http://www.tandf.co.uk/journals

Ethics content was enhanced according to the template that was developed (Table 6.1). Where there was a match between the desired level of content and the analysis of that content within the problems, no changes were made to the scenarios. Changes were implemented in the other instances. Learning that occurred in the small group setting was complemented by large group sessions scattered across the program. These sessions addressed ethical theory, research, assessment of personal and class core values, and included clinical scenarios and discussion of some of the twelve ethical issues.

While the students have a significant level of autonomy in identifying, researching and discussing learning questions related to each health care problem, the tutor facilitates and assists in guiding their learning. Tutors are provided with written tutor guides to make them aware of the key concepts and knowledge areas for each health care problem. With the implementation of the ethics content, tutor guides were adapted and tutor training provided.

After each tutorial, students research the learning questions that are identified and return to discuss and synthesize the content at the next session. Students readily become skilled in searching and appraising the literature but this tends to be limited to

Table 6.1. Ethical issues relevant to physical therapy practice

Ethical issue	Definition	Depth of learning within curriculum[a]	Placement of learning with curriculum
1. Informed consent	The right of a capable person to choose what will happen to his/her body or mind. Age may be applicable in some jurisdictions	Greater	Term 1
2. Truth-telling	Duty to keep the client informed and to honestly answer his/her questions and/or refer client to appropriate health care professional	Greater	Term 2
3. Privacy/confidentiality	Collection, use and disclosure of client's identifiable information only with client consent	Greater	Across all six terms
4. Quality of life	Right to a satisfying and meaningful existence from the client's perspective	Greater	Term 5
5. Allocation of scarce resources	Balancing duties of justice and fairness for client with those for the payer and/or society	Greater	Term 4
6. Professional collegiality	Fidelity and respect for your profession and other health care professionals while ensuring client's rights take precedence	Greater	Term 6
7. Advocacy for client	Supporting the interests of the client	Moderate	Term 3
8. Societal well-being	Duty to the common good as a therapist and citizen	Moderate	No decision
9. Respect for individual differences	Principle of equality and of an individual's dignity and value. No systematic or individual bias based on gender, race, culture, etc.	Moderate	Term 3
10. Experimental treatment	Informing clients about experimental treatments (purpose, risk, benefits) and ensuring informed consent for participation with right to withdraw	Superficial	No decision
11. Organ transplantation/donation	Procuring and allocating tissues for transplantation	Superficial	Term 4
12. End of life decisions	Decisions about initiating, continuing, or discontinuing treatment when a person is dying	Superficial	Term 4

[a] Superficial depth = knowledge/comprehension; moderate depth = application; greater depth = analysis/synthesis

Adapted from Geddes et al. (1998, 1999, 2004)

the health care domain. Given that much of the literature on ethics is within the social science domains, and that students have time limitations, the Physiotherapy Program conducted an extensive literature review on each of the twelve ethical issues and selected the most appropriate citations linking ethics and rehabilitation. These were compiled into a resource manual along with a description of each ethical issue (Geddes et al. 1998, 1999).

The final step in any curriculum revision is the evaluation of the process and of the content changes. Process evaluation occurred through dialogue with faculty. The impact of content changes was evaluated through an interprofessional research study by both programs and is described below.

The integration of ethics content into the bachelor-level physiotherapy curriculum was a dynamic and stepwise process. When the physiotherapy program was changed to a professional masters degree [MSc(PT)], many of the health care problems and the linked ethics content were carried forward; however, changes occurred in the overall curriculum design reflecting changes in the health care environment and physiotherapy profession in the twenty-first century. Thus, the Program is broadening the ethics stream to address the "professionalization" of our students. Ethics is an important aspect, along with reflective practice, professional behaviors, and communication skills.

Ethics Education in the Occupational Therapy Program

In the Occupational Therapy Program at McMaster University, students choose to study four or five problems each term from a wide selection of scenarios. Each tutorial group is encouraged to explore their chosen problem by selecting a theoretical model. This gives the students a framework for their learning in which they identify occupational performance issues and determine appropriate means of assessment and intervention.

Prior to a review of the ethics education component in the Program in the mid 1990s, a few ethics initiatives were already in place. All students received a copy of a small booklet entitled *Introduction to Ethical Decision-Making in Health Care* (McMaster University 1993) published by a committee within the Faculty of Health Sciences. This booklet offered a brief introduction to ethics theory and decision-making models developed for health care professionals, primarily in medicine and nursing. It was intended that these theoretical models be used in the problems that had been devoted to ethics in the Occupational Therapy Program. These problems alluded to overt ethical dilemmas for which the College of Occupational Therapists of Ontario offered clear direction. Large group seminar sessions reinforced ethics learning.

Work done by Brockett (1997) was the catalyst for the review of the ethics content in the Occupational Therapy Program. In her doctoral dissertation, she concluded that rules and regulations are inadequate as a means of controlling the excesses of professionalism. Professional self-interest and the desire for status and power make it profitable for practitioners to keep clients in a subservient position where compliance is expected. She suggested that trustworthiness, as an inherent feature of ethical behavior, depends more on building relationships of authentic respect. Such respect invites mutual recognition of the cultures, values, and traditions with which each person is identified, a sharing of those that they hold in common, and an awareness of their differences and limitations. This approach is consistent with the client-centered practice of occupational therapy (Canadian Association of Occupational Therapists 1997). It appears to call for "moral sensitivity," one element in Rest's Four Component Model of Moral Behavior (Rest 1994 p. 23) described as "the awareness of how our actions affect other people."

The faculty agreed that extra emphasis on building moral sensitivity would be given to the ethics education program. In the years that followed this decision, students were invited to attend an ethics session in each term. These sessions had an emphasis on morality and promoted the "art" of ethical decision making through the building of a "big picture" preliminary to identifying the ethical issues that might affect clinical practice. Much of the time was spent in unpacking and understanding the ethical issues associated with difficult situations that students had encountered in their clinical fieldwork.

As the ethics emphasis gained recognition, there was an attempt to offer ethical guidelines to tutors through detailed analyses of the problems offered to students in tutorials, supplemented by discussion at tutors' meetings. This required an acceptance of the premise that all problems involving relationships have a moral component. Some of the curricular units offered more opportunities to raise moral issues in large group seminars than others. For example, in the unit on "aging," social and professional responses toward death and dying and palliative care became a topic for discussion, as did the matter of individual rights and community responsibilities.

Initially, there was very little structure to the ethics education curriculum in the occupational therapy program. This was partly because student participation was voluntary. Gradually, however, it became an accepted component of the curriculum, expanding to include an interprofessional session with physiotherapy students. Ultimately, this increased recognition of ethics led to support for ethics education as a core theme in the development of the masters entry-level occupational therapy [MSc(OT)] curriculum.

The MSc(OT) program curriculum is organized within a framework that incorporates three constructs: Person-Environment-Occupation; Professional Preparation and Development; and Transition to Practice. There are four curricular threads: simplicity to complexity; unifaceted to multifaceted; wellness to illness; and local to global. Broad categories of issues such as ethics, legal implications of practice, and policy planning are interwoven throughout the curriculum. Each of the six terms has a particular focus while learning is encouraged through inquiry, reflection, and evidence-based practice.

The ethics curriculum (Table 6.2) is introduced through a formal Inquiry class each term and applied through the problem-based tutorials, the Professional Roles and Experiential Practicum, and in assignments. For example, the Inquiry class in the first year focuses on the students' perceptions of "self" within the wider society and how that person can influence change, as well as be changed, by interactions with others. In the second year, the focus moves to concepts of community and collaboration between and among groups to effect changes within systems and institutions. In the tutorial course, tutors are asked to facilitate ethics inquiry through the use of questions worded to elicit the contextual picture of the relationships involved in any problem scenario. Professional Roles and Experiential Practicum classes build the skills and strategies needed for increased personal awareness in relationships; in one term this is accomplished by having students write "relational response" papers in which they reflect on their experiences and the connections that they have recognized in all three courses. Scholarly paper assignments always include ethical issues as a choice and one of five questions in a Clinical Reasoning Examination given at the conclusion of term 2 requires recall of the ethics content to that point.

Table 6.2. Preliminary ethics content of MSc(OT) program

Focus of term	Focus of ethics content[a]
1. Wellness, health and occupation – looking at the relationship between these concepts, the need for, and aims of occupational therapy	"Doing ethics" – what is involved? Building the big picture of ethical issues Questions that should be asked Organizing individual and professional options in a way that reveals the nature of ethical choices Clinical practice assignment – record situations of disease related to behavior
2. Person, environment, and occupation – assessment, interpreting the interaction of a person with his/her environment and the factors that may be contributing to occupational dysfunction	"Becoming self-aware" How our behavior is perceived by others Assessing our own knowledge and capacity to make ethical decisions that respect the different perspectives of legal and moral concerns with which we are identified
3. Disability, development, and occupation – intervention – recognizing the impact of disability upon occupation and exploring options for improved performance	"When there is disagreement" Informed consent and risk management Dilemmas and decision-making models
4. Youth and the development of self – the challenges involved in nurturing meaningful occupations as children and young people with varying capacities mature in a complex society	"Concepts of community" Ethics teams and dissent Competence and supportive, collaborative learning environments
5. Adulthood and disability – the challenges involved in facilitating occupational adaptation among adults as they age in a society that is in a constant state of change	"Nurturing community responsibility" Changes that respect the individual rights and identities of people as they age and die
6. Complexities of contemporary practice – transition to professional practice	Transitions from being the student/client to becoming the facilitator/clinical expert – ethical ambiguity and ethical maturity

[a] Ethical perspectives are primarily presented within the Inquiry and Integration large group sessions. Guidelines for tutors offer questions to assist students in enlarging upon the ethical focus of the term and provide a connection between the large group content and small group discussion

Most recently, faculty members have recognized that the ethics content being taught in the new curriculum has strong connections with spirituality and culture. Spirituality is seen as the subjective and qualitative meaning that comes from within and influences a person's sense of being. Culture is understood to be the lived experience of "being" held in common with another, or others, which influences behavior. The founding question of ethics "How should I conduct my life in the presence of other lives?" (Seedhouse 1998 p. 8) calls for behavior that honors personal spiritual values and the cultural experiences shared with others. This new understanding fits well with the Person-Environment-Occupation model (Fig. 6.3; Law et al. 1996) where occupa-

In addition, the two disciplines meet together in large group seminars to discuss the students' professional transition into their respective professions. One of these sessions has a focus on the legislation that affects practice and another gives the floor to the regulatory colleges. Yet another considers the ethics of professionalism and revisits the concepts of law and morality. The students are also invited to reflect on the ways in which their perspectives and behaviors have been influenced and changed by their programs.

Lessons Learned

Faculty Involvement

In our experience, the development and inclusion of ethics in the curriculum requires commitment by the faculty, a champion to spearhead the curriculum design, implementation and evaluation, and a subgroup of faculty to assist in this process. In problem-based learning, with integration of content within and across terms of study, all faculty need to "buy-in" to any changes in the curricular content. Faculty must share in deciding what, where, and how to include specific content. To most effectively accomplish this we have found that one faculty member with skill and expertise in the topic is required to provide leadership and direction for incorporating ethics into the curriculum.

Establishment of Learning Objectives

It is essential that learning objectives (knowledge, skills, and behaviors) for ethics in the curriculum are clear. What do you wish to accomplish, what do you wish to include, and how will you evaluate outcomes? Ethics education must move beyond simply including codes of ethics, rules and legal requirements, and/or knowledge of ethical theories. At McMaster University, both programs have focused on the moral judgment, sensitivity, and reasoning of students in the context of clinical decision making. While this includes understanding necessary rules and norms for practice, it requires systematic reflection on one's personal values, beliefs, and behaviors as well as those of colleagues, clients, the profession, and society, appreciation of the effects of one's actions upon others, linking ethical decision making with clinical decision making, and the ability to defend the choices made.

Maintaining and Adapting Content

Once the learning objectives have been determined, sustaining the ethics content over time is an ongoing challenge. It is not a static situation. The faculty, tutors, and learning resources fluctuate, time and financial resources exert pressure, and new evidence needs to be searched and appraised. This requires constant adaptation of the ethics curriculum.

The clinical context also influences ethics content. Educators need to be aware of the different experiences of occupational therapists and physiotherapists in the clinical setting and the ethical issues that are being encountered by students and clinicians.

Barnitt (1998) compared the ethical dilemmas encountered by both professions and found that of the seven themes identified by occupational therapists and the six themes identified by physiotherapists, four were shared between the two groups. However, the frequency of encountering these issues varied widely between the professions. Furthermore, the most common practice area for ethical issues for occupational therapists was mental health while for physiotherapists it was shared between respiratory, neurological, orthopedic and surgical settings (Barnitt 1998).

The health care systems within which occupational therapy and physiotherapy students are trained also influences the ethical issues they will encounter. Barnitt (1998) from the United Kingdom, Geddes et al. (1998) from Canada, and Triezenberg (1997) from the United States each identified ethical issues experienced by physiotherapists in practice. The only common theme reported by the authors was allocation of scarce resources. Some themes such as informed consent and truth telling were shared between two of the countries and some themes such as product endorsement and maintenance of competence were found only in one.

Students do identify ethical issues in the clinical setting. Analysis of journals written by a class of physiotherapy students during their second six-week clinical placement, indicated that students frequently encountered ethical issues (Geddes et al. 2004). Fifty-three of the 56 students wrote about ethical issues in a total of 280 journal entries. From these entries, the researchers identified six ethical themes and were able to categorize them as major or minor based on the frequency with which the themes arose. The major themes were respect for the uniqueness of the individual, professionalism, and professional collegiality. The minor themes were allocation of resources, advocacy for the client, society, and/or health policy, and informed consent. Although not studied formally, the experience of students in the Occupational Therapy Program supports these findings.

Process and Format for Ethics Education

The process and format for ethics education employed in both programs at McMaster University has reflected the uniqueness of each discipline. Barnitt and Partridge (1997) suggested that differences exist between occupational therapists and physiotherapists in their ethical reasoning styles. Occupational therapists were more likely to use a narrative style of reasoning, emphasizing the social context and history of the current problem and describing several parallel themes at once. Physiotherapists on the other hand, used a procedural style, focused around the diagnosis and the implications for treatment and described the situation in a more linear fashion (Barnitt and Partridge 1997). Furthermore, as mentioned earlier in the chapter, the two professions may demonstrate differing personality types. Lysack et al. (2001), using the Myers-Briggs Type Indicator, suggested that physiotherapists were more likely to be "judging" and occupational therapists were more likely to be "perceiving." The authors hypothesized that the possible reasons for these findings related to the different job functions, the historical development and guiding principles, and the public perceptions of each profession. The work of Hardigan and Cohen (1998) supported Lysack et al.'s (2001) findings for physiotherapists, but found that occupational therapists were equally likely to be "judging" or "perceiving."

This evidence suggests that educators should approach ethics education differently for student occupational therapists compared to student physiotherapists, but it begs the following questions. Should the approach within the curricula mirror the ethical reasoning styles and predominant personality type of each profession or should each curriculum encourage its students to expand their thinking to other reasoning styles and personality types? Are the different reasoning styles the result of the professionalization process or a reflection of the self-selection process in which students choose either profession? Our research has shown that our ethics education process, which mirrored the reasoning and personality styles of each profession, did result in significantly improved moral judgment over the course of the students' training in occupational therapy and physiotherapy. Clearly further inquiry is warranted.

Role of the Tutor

Within the small group tutorial sessions, students have substantial autonomy regarding their learning choices, but the role of tutor is essential for providing guidance and feedback. As in other areas of study, however, the body of literature on health care ethics is burgeoning and it is a challenge for tutors to keep abreast of the most current literature. Also, tutors may not feel skilled in facilitating discussion on ethics. Therefore, ongoing tutor training is essential within the problem-based learning context even though tutors may have varying levels of interest and/or time to participate in additional resource sessions. At the minimum, key information and references should be provided within the tutor guide for the health care problem.

Interprofessional Education

Given the increasingly interprofessional context of health care and the blurring in the scopes of practice of health care professions, providing interprofessional learning in ethics is highly desirable. Students need to have the opportunity to develop their relationships with colleagues and gain an appreciation of both shared and differing ethical perspectives.

While we have had some success in interprofessional education events related to ethics, we have also experienced several barriers to implementation. In order to be successful, those interested in developing interprofessional activities must address the following:

- The differing pedagogical formats for addressing ethics content

- The timing of content across the various programs

- The commitment of the various departments to interprofessional events

- The differing scheduling of students in the health care programs

- The accessibility to physical spaces for large group sessions as well as "breakouts" rooms for small groups

Perhaps most importantly, the sessions need to be perceived as valuable by the students for them to attend. Student involvement in the development and execution of the events enhances student participation.

Student Barriers to Learning Ethics

Students may not value ethics content, viewing it a "soft" content compared to other core content (e.g., pathology, anatomy) and thus place less emphasis for learning on this topic (Solomon and Geddes 2000). In their study of tutorial groups completing one health care problem, Solomon and Geddes (2000) found that 12 percent of the tutorial time was spent discussing ethical issues and that at least two-thirds of the time the students initiated the discussion. The researchers concluded physiotherapy "students did make choices to pursue learning related to ethics and were able to discuss relevant learning issues adequately" (Solomon and Geddes 2000 p. 285). However, they identified several barriers that impacted on the students' learning.

> **》** Students' ... lack of language and knowledge related to ethics made it difficult for them to appreciate the nature of their discussions and to define ethically related learning issues. This, in conjunction with competing content, and the perception that it is difficult to access appropriate literature, may have resulted in the students' lower priorization of ethics. The lack of clinical experience also seems to create a barrier for students in their appreciation of the importance of ethics in health care practice. (Solomon and Geddes 2000 p. 285)

Conclusions

Ethics is an accepted part of both the Occupational Therapy and Physiotherapy Programs at McMaster University. It has undergone development and change over time as the needs of each program have evolved. Both programs began the process of explicitly addressing ethics in their bachelor-level programs in the mid 1990s. Within the problem-based pedagogical foundation, the ethics content was integrated as a stream topic across each two-year program. With the transition to the MSc(OT) and MSc(PT) programs in 2000, ethics has become a rich core of the new occupational therapy curriculum along with spirituality and culture and is being integrated with professionalization in the physiotherapy curriculum with the goal of developing caring, reflective practitioners. Though both programs have undertaken different approaches to implementing ethics education in their curricula, our research shows that the moral judgment of both occupational therapy and physiotherapy students at McMaster University significantly improves during the course of their training.

Acknowledgements

The authors wish to acknowledge our colleagues who have shared with us in the development and implementation of the ethics streams in both curricula – Ron Dick BHScOT, Professional Associate, School of Rehabilitation Science, McMaster University and Occupational Therapist, St Joseph's Healthcare, Hamilton, Ontario; Elspeth Finch BScP&OT, MHSc, Associate Professor, School of Rehabilitation Science, McMaster University; Karen Graham BPE, BED, BHScPT, Professional Associate, School of Rehabilitation Science, McMaster University and Physical Therapist, Hamilton Health Sciences, Hamilton, Ontario; and Dr. Helene Larin PhD, PT, Assistant Professor, School of Nursing and School of Rehabilitation Science, McMaster University.

6

References

Barnitt RE (1993) 'Deeply troubling questions': the teaching of ethics in undergraduate courses. Br J Occup Ther 56:401–406

Barnitt R (1998) Ethical dilemmas in occupational therapy and physical therapy: a survey of practitioners in the UK National Health Service. J Med Ethics 24:193–199

Barnitt R, Partridge C (1997) Ethical reasoning in physical therapy and occupational therapy. Physiother Res Int 2:178–192

Brockett M (1996) Ethics, moral reasoning and professional virtue in occupational therapy education. Can J Occup Ther 63:197–205

Brockett M (1997) Building trustworthy relationships: a reconstruction of ethics education for the health care professions. Dissertation University of Toronto, ON

Canadian Association of Occupational Therapists (1997) Enabling occupation: an occupational therapy perspective. CAOT/ACE, Ottawa, ON

De Casterlé BD, Janssen PJ, Grypdonck M (1996) The relationship between education and ethical behaviour of nursing students. West J Nurs Res 18:330–350

e-Laws: Ontario Statutes and Regulations. http://www.e-laws.gov.on.ca/. Retrieved 20 July 2004

Finley C, Goldstein MS (1991) Curriculum survey: ethical and legal instruction: a report from the APTA Department of Education and the APTA Judicial Committee. J Phys Ther Educ 5:60–64

Geddes EL (1998) Ethics, moral reasoning and professional virtue in physiotherapy education in Canada. Physiother Can 50(suppl):13

Geddes EL, Finch E, Larin H, Janson R, Taylor M (1998) Ethics in physiotherapy practice: determining key issues for student learning. Physiother Can 50(suppl):13

Geddes EL, Finch E, Larin H (1999) Ethical issues relevant to physical therapy. School of Rehabilitation Science, McMaster University, Hamilton, ON

Geddes EL, Wessel J, Williams R (2004) Ethical issues identified by physical therapy students during clinical placements. Physiother Theory Pract 20:17–29

Geddes EL, Finch E, Graham K (2005) Ethical choices: a moral and legal template for health care practice. Physiother Can 57:113–121

Goldie J, Schwartz L, McConnachie A, Morrison J (2001) Impact of a new course on students' potential behaviour on encountering ethical dilemmas. Med Educ 35:295–302

Gronlund NE (1985) Stating objectives for classroom instruction, 3rd edn. Macmillan, New York, NY

Hardigan PC, Cohen SR (1998) Comparison of personality styles between students enrolled in osteopathic, medical, pharmacy, physical therapy, physician assistant, and occupational therapy programs. Med Educ 98:637–641

Kelley M (2002) The meanings of professional life: teaching across the health professions. J Med Philos 27:475–491

Krawczyk RM (1997) Teaching ethics: effect on moral development. Nurs Ethics 4:57–65

Law M, Cooper BA, Strong S, Stewart D, Rigby P, Letts L (1996) The person-environment-occupation model: a transactive approach to occupational performance. Can J Occup Ther 63:9–23

Lysack C, McNevin N, Dunleavy K (2001) Job choice and personality: a profile of Michigan occupational and physical therapists. J Allied Health 30:75–82

McMaster University, Faculty of Health Sciences (1993) Introduction to ethical decision-making in health care. McMaster University, Hamilton, ON

Patenaude J, Niyonsenga T, Fafard D (2003) Changes in students' moral development during medical school: a cohort study. Can Med Assoc J 168:840–844

Privacy Commissioner of Canada (2004) The personal information protection and electronic documents act. http://www.privcom.gc.ca/legislation/02_06_01_e.asp. Retrieved 2 Feb 2004

Rest JR (1994) Background: theory and research. In: Rest JR, Narváez D (eds) Moral development in the professions: psychology and applied ethics. Erlbaum, Hillsdale, NJ, pp 1–26

Rest JR, Narváez D (1994) Moral development in the professions: psychology and applied ethics. Erlbaum, Hillsdale, NJ

Rest J, Thoma SJ, Narváez D, Bebeau M (1996) Alchemy and beyond: indexing the defining issues test. Center for the Study of Ethical Development, University of Minnesota, Minneapolis

Rest J, Narváez D, Bebeau M, Thoma SJ (1999) Postconventional moral thinking: a neo-kohlbergian approach. Erlbaum, Mahwah, NJ

Saarinen-Rahiika H, Binkley JM (1998) Problem-based learning in physical therapy: a review of the literature and overview of the McMaster University experience. Phys Ther 78:195–206

Seedhouse D (1998) Ethics: the heart of health care. Wiley, Chichester

Solomon P, Geddes EL (2000) Influences of physiotherapy students' choices to pursue learning related to ethics in a problem-based curriculum. Physiother Can 52:279–285

Solomon P, Geddes EL (2001) A systematic process for content review in a problem-based learning curriculum. Med Teach 23:556–560

Solomon P, Blumberg P, Shehata A (1992) The influence of a patient's age on problem-based tutorial discussion. Acad Med 67:S31–S33

Swisher LL (2002) A retrospective analysis of ethics knowledge in physical therapy (1970–2000). Phys Ther 82:692–706

ten Have HAMJ (1995) Ethics in the clinic: a comparison of two Dutch teaching programmes. Med Educ 29:34–38

Triezenberg HL (1996) The identification of ethical issues in physical therapy practice. Phys Ther 76:1097–1108

6

Chapter 7

Interprofessional Education

Penny Salvatori, Patricia Solomon

Contents

7

In 1978, the World Health Organization (WHO) identified interprofessional education (IPE) as an important component of primary health care. In Canada, the Ottawa Charter for Health Promotion (1986) called for IPE to meet changing societal needs. A statement from the Ontario Chairs of Family Medicine and the Council of Ontario University Programs in Nursing also addressed the need for collaborative interdisciplinary teams in the context of primary health care reform in Ontario and further suggested that interdisciplinary education should be mandatory for all health sciences students (Pringle et al. 2000). Tryssenaar et al. (1996) reported similar support for IPE amongst occupational therapy and physiotherapy programs across Canada. Most recently, the Romanow (2002) report on the Future of Health Care in Canada suggested IPE and collaboration are "essential to achieving effective delivery of health care" (Romanow 2002 p. 109). Clearly, external pressures are driving the renewed interest in IPE and the recent flurry of activity in the decade since 1995.

Since the WHO declaration, various health professional education programs throughout the world have attempted to introduce IPE into their curricula. Some have been more successful than others. The philosophical argument is clear and widely accepted: IPE at the pre-licensure level will lead to improved interprofessional collaboration in practice and ultimately improved health outcomes for patients. However, there is little agreement in the literature regarding what teaching strategies are most effective, when best to introduce IPE into professional programs, and how much intervention is required. In addition, several barriers and challenges to implementing IPE have been identified. These include timetable conflicts, lack of institutional support, rigid academic hierarchies, negative faculty attitudes, and costs (Erickson et al. 1998; Larson 1995). It is clear that the traditional "silo" approach to education provides little or no opportunity for students to become familiar with the values, roles, and expertise of other health professionals (Bainbridge and Matthews 1996; Clark 1997; Cleary and Howell 2003; Irvine et al. 2002). Therefore, as Singleton and Green-Hernandez (1998 p. 5) have suggested, it is unrealistic to expect "unknown neighbors" to be colleagues.

While the literature identifies common challenges to implementing IPE, the question of effectiveness of IPE remains largely unanswered. Hammick (2000), however, is quick to point out that lack of evidence of effectiveness does not necessarily mean that IPE is ineffective. Good quality effectiveness studies are lacking. Unfortunately, most of the literature is descriptive, very few studies have employed a rigorous design or included an evaluation component, and few replication studies have been done.

A systematic review was conducted to answer the question "Does interprofessional education benefit patients?" (Barr et al. 1999 p. 107). After reviewing 1,042 abstracts and evaluating 86 papers, none were found to meet the inclusion criteria, and a negative report was filed in the Cochrane Library. Based on this work, Hammick (2000) compiled a list of potential outcomes for IPE evaluation purposes: (a) learner reaction/satisfaction, (b) changes in attitudes/perceptions, (c) changes in knowledge and skills, (d) changes in practice behavior, (e) changes in organizational culture and structure, and (f) improved health outcomes. Although not labeled as such, the above list appears to be somewhat hierarchical in terms of the ease of both implementing and measuring change as a result of IPE interventions.

In 2001, Cooper et al. conducted another systematic review of evidence to support interprofessional learning for health professional students. On the basis of 30 articles that met their inclusion criteria, they reported positive outcomes related to changes in knowledge, skills, attitudes, and beliefs, although effects on professional practice behavior were not found (Cooper et al. 2001). Barr (2001) also discussed the emerging evidence and concluded that "interprofessional education can, in favourable circumstances and in different ways, contribute to improving collaboration in practice" (Barr 2001 p. 25).

In 2002, Freeth et al. conducted another review which allowed for a wider range of research methodologies and also broadened the outcomes of interest beyond patient benefits to include the impact on learners and organizations. They reported that fewer than 30 percent of studies focused on pre-licensure students and most often the IPE location was a service delivery setting rather than the university setting. Based on a small set of higher quality studies, Freeth et al. concluded that some evidence exists to support improved learner attitudes/perceptions, knowledge, and skills following an IPE intervention; however, they also reiterated the need for further research using more rigorous longitudinal and before-after designs as well as qualitative methods.

The challenge to educators is to work together to cross disciplinary boundaries and overcome institutional barriers in order to design, implement, and evaluate shared learning experiences at the pre-licensure level in order to prepare our students with the requisite knowledge, attitudes, and skills required for interprofessional collaboration in practice.

Before describing the efforts at McMaster University to meet this challenge, it is important to clearly define IPE. Hammick distinguishes between IPE which she defines as "learning together to promote collaborative practice" (Hammick 2000 p. 461) and multiprofessional education (MPE) which she refers to as "learning together for whatever reason" (Hammick 2000 p. 461). Zwarenstein et al. (2002) have expanded on Hammick's definition and suggest that "an IPE intervention occurs when members of more than one health and/or social care profession learn interactively together, for the explicit purpose of improving inter-professional collaboration and/or the health/well-being of patients/clients" (Zwarenstein et al. 2002 p. 3). The above will serve as our working definitions as we proceed to recount our personal experiences.

Interprofessional Education in Rehabilitation Science at McMaster University

The history of IPE education for occupational therapy and physiotherapy students in the Hamilton area begins back in the early 1980s when professional training programs were offered at the diploma level at Mohawk College. This section of the chapter will use a chronological approach to describe some of the IPE initiatives offered from that time to the present, highlighting key features of the students' learning experiences and the lessons learned for faculty along the way. More recent IPE learning experiences that were formally evaluated are described in detail.

In the Beginning – Mohawk College to McMaster University 1980–1990

The importance of interprofessional learning was recognized twenty-five years ago when the occupational therapy and physiotherapy programs were housed at Mohawk College in Hamilton. The first IPE initiative was a two-day human sexuality workshop with lectures and small group tutorials offered to the occupational therapy and physiotherapy students at Mohawk College and the nursing, medical, and social work students at McMaster University. Faculty tutors were drawn from Mohawk College and McMaster University which, in itself, represented a truly interprofessional collaborative effort. Over time, all of the education programs began to integrate the sexuality content into the core curriculum and this optional workshop was discontinued.

The success of this event prompted the development of several IPE one-day workshops for McMaster University health sciences students on topics such as gender sensitivity, teamwork in health care, community health care, legal issues, and palliative care. Attendance was optional and therefore sporadic; however, all of the workshops were evaluated highly by those who participated. Each of the workshops relied on a faculty champion to keep the initiative going. As one might expect, as the champions departed or gave up their role, most of the IPE workshops were discontinued over time. Only the Palliative Care workshop remains an ongoing event today because of the existence of committed faculty and student planning group which organizes this workshop on an annual basis. Our experience suggests that these optional and isolated special events are difficult to organize and costly in terms of faculty time and resources.

In the mid 1980s when the BHSc degree completion course was put in place at McMaster for the Mohawk diploma graduates, the Population Health course offered in the School of Nursing became a required course for the occupational therapy and physiotherapy students. Students in Kinesiology and post-degree Nursing also attended this course which was valued highly by both students and faculty. Unfortunately, much to the disappointment of the Nursing faculty, when the Mohawk diploma programs and the BHSc degree completion program were phased out and two new second-degree baccalaureate programs were implemented at McMaster in 1990, the new curricula did not include Population Health as a core course.

The BHSc OT and BHSc PT Programs 1990–2000

Although our experiences in the 1980s demonstrated that attendance was a problem if the IPE experience was not mandatory, the positive evaluations of the initiatives and our strong belief in the importance of collaborative teamwork led to an increased commitment to IPE. With the development of the new BHSc Occupational Therapy and Physiotherapy Programs, there was a deliberate attempt to integrate IPE opportunities into the required courses. In the first semester, the Inquiry Seminar course focused broadly on health issues. Occupational therapy and physiotherapy students worked in small groups to investigate problem scenarios, prepare for large group discussions, and collaborate on a written assignment. While other courses in the occupational therapy program shared the same broad focus as an introduction to the profession, the concurrent physiotherapy courses were more narrowly focused on human biology and musculoskeletal disorders. Thus it was not surprising that the feedback from the physiotherapy students indicated dissatisfaction with the lack of fit with the course content and learning objectives. As a result, the combined Inquiry Seminar course was discontinued after three years.

Combined occupational therapy and physiotherapy courses in the final semester of study were more successful as both groups of students were able to appreciate the relevance of the content. A "Management Skills" course was developed to prepare graduating students for the transition to the real world of clinical practice. Students were required to work in interprofessional groups to prepare seminars on a variety of topics such as the funding of the health care system, avoiding professional burnout, and program evaluation. The research course in this semester also provided opportunities for occupational therapy and physiotherapy students to work together on a research project. All of these IPE learning experiences were valued highly by both students and faculty and thus remained in place until the baccalaureate programs were replaced by entry-level masters programs in 2000.

In 1991, the Faculty of Health Sciences formed a committee with a mandate to enhance IPE. The committee was responsible for overseeing the IPE workshops and was also challenged to develop new IPE opportunities. Despite many creative ideas such as interprofessional research projects and community-based projects, timetable conflicts posed a major barrier and there was a lack of faculty commitment to change the status quo. It was also clear that the players around that table did not value IPE to the same extent and not all were prepared to champion the cause within their own faculty group. As a result, this committee was disbanded after five years.

Recognizing the inherent scheduling difficulties in organizing IPE initiatives in the academic setting, several champions developed successful initiatives in the clinical setting. In 1993, a local Community Health Center offered a new community-based IPE clinical experience to students (van der Horst et al. 1995). The educational model consisted of small group discussion with some didactic instruction and problem-based learning. Groups of six to eight students from nursing, medicine, occupational therapy, physiotherapy, and social work programs met with two faculty facilitators for a three-hour session each week for eight consecutive weeks during their clinical placements. Learning objectives focused on various aspects of team functioning which served as the topics for weekly discussions: team dynamics; role issues and professional values; collaboration and conflict; communication, leadership and power; client-centered goal-oriented care and consumerism. As part of the project, the students shared their knowledge of interprofessional team care for the elderly through a panel presentation to a group of consumers. Formal evaluation of the project indicated that students experienced new learning in relation to each other's roles and team functioning. They enjoyed the IPE experience, especially sharing diverse opinions and problem-solving together. There were unanticipated benefits for the clinicians who participated in the sessions (i.e., professional development related to team functioning and conflict resolution), and improved communication between the health center, community agencies, and university programs was noted. Although plans were described to expand the project to eight groups of students in the following year and to conduct a six- to eight-month follow-up evaluation (van der Horst et al. 1995), it is unknown if these plans were ever realized. The IPE experience has not been offered at the Center for many years.

Another unique IPE experience in the clinical setting was a team placement at a regional geriatric hospital (Richardson et al. 1999). In this project, a group of students from occupational therapy, physiotherapy, nursing, social work, and therapeutic recreation worked together as a student team in the Geriatric Day Hospital for a six-week period. Despite numerous attempts, no medical student was recruited. The clinicians on the team acted as preceptors and provided student supervision. Two of the investigators ran weekly two-hour problem-based tutorials focused on interprofessional teams, roles, communication, client-centered practice, conflict management, leadership, and accountability. The Interprofessional Perception Scale was used to examine how students view their own profession, view other professionals, and their beliefs on how other professionals view them. Results revealed no statistically significant difference between the experimental group and the control group at pre- or post-test. While 80 percent agreed that health professionals in general are competent and highly ethical, and that good relationships with other professionals are possible, 70 percent felt other professions were more territorial than their own. Exit interviews of student participants indicated they appreciated the support they provided for one another in terms of feeling comfortable and taking risks in the larger team. Students also reported increased knowledge in relation to professional roles and team functioning. Finally, the Team Observation Protocol results suggested that students were able to share information and interact jointly with clients in a collaborative way. Given the positive learning outcomes, it is unfortunate that this IPE experience was discontinued after the pilot phase was completed. Like the project at the community health center described above, it would appear that time-limited funding created a major barrier in terms of long-term sustainability.

The MSc OT and MSc PT Programs 2000–Present

When the curricula for the new MSc Occupational Therapy and Physiotherapy Programs were being developed there was another deliberate attempt to integrate IPE into the final unit of academic study. A seminar/lecture series covered topics related to the transition to professional practice such as establishing a private practice, developing proposals for new clinical programs or professional roles, interacting within the legal system, and professional ethics. Unlike the previous course in the BHSc Programs, this course was based more on multiprofessional educational principles which serve to bring students together in the same classroom but do not require any interaction or collaboration. Nonetheless, student feedback has been positive.

A series of interprofessional tutorials and skills workshops were also designed to provide an opportunity for occupational therapy and physiotherapy students to develop an understanding of the professional roles and responsibilities of each profession in clinical practice. There was a strong emphasis on issues of teamwork and communication. Small group tutorials, with equal distribution of occupational therapy and physiotherapy students, worked together on three problem-based scenarios related to a patient living with chronic pain, one with severe burns, and another who had an above-knee amputation. Faculty tutors were drawn from both professions.

Students also participated in complementary skills workshops which focused on the clinical assessment and treatment aspects related to the clinical scenarios they were studying in the tutorial. The skills workshops were designed as a series of stations related to assessment and management, through which students rotated with other members of their tutorial group. For example, one station examined functional assessment of an amputee patient, while another station examined assessments related to impairment in an amputee patient, such as skin integrity, sensation, and muscle strength. Students were encouraged to work in pairs as an occupational therapy and physiotherapy "team" in order to learn the various assessment and treatment techniques from their colleagues. This initiative posed several challenges. The occupational therapy and physiotherapy students had developed different styles and methods of approaching the tutorial process as there was some variation in the programmatic approach. Additionally, the physiotherapy students tended to focus on the pathophysiology and clinical features of the condition, while the occupational therapy students focused more globally on client-centered problems and goals. While some students were able to see the differences as a way of working as a team to make decisions, others simply saw this as a deterrent to learning the content of the tutorial problem. This was particularly the case for physiotherapy students who were worried about profession-specific content related to their pending licensing examinations. Scheduling logistics also influenced the extent to which students valued the tutorial process. The interprofessional tutorials were in addition to the occupational therapy students' regular timetable, thus they saw this event as an "add-on" and did not value the sessions to the same extent as the physiotherapy students.

Not surprisingly, student feedback of the initiative was mixed. Feedback indicated that students liked the fact that the tutorial and skills workshops were complementary. Students felt that some myths about the professions had been dispelled as a result of their experience. Other students failed to see the value in spending time together learning about the other profession and felt that the tutorials would be of greater benefit if they focused on profession-specific issues.

This IPE initiative has been modified since it was implemented three years ago and will be maintained as part of the core curriculum. Objectives are now clearly focused on IPE issues such as communication, understanding each other's roles, and teamwork. For example, problem scenarios have been revised to highlight issues of team functioning in addition to disease-specific content. Tutorials for both occupational therapy and physiotherapy are integrated into the schedule and no longer perceived by occupational therapy students as an add-on. Both groups of students are now examined on the content of laboratories and tutorials.

In 2000, a new Interdisciplinary Student Council was formed in the Faculty of Health Sciences by a visionary group of students. The group saw its mandate as providing both social and academic events to promote interaction among health sciences students. This Council has become stronger over the years with student representatives from all education programs. A faculty member was appointed to the committee for liaison purposes. The Council participates in the annual Student Welcome day in September and sponsors at least one social and one academic event in each semester. The Council is currently actively involved in planning additional IPE events such as a journal club and perhaps a community clinic.

Also in 2000, the Ministry of Health provided new funding to Health Sciences North to implement and evaluate new IPE initiatives in Northern Ontario (P. Salvatori, S. Berry, and K. Eva, submitted for publication). McMaster University partnered with Health Sciences North in Thunder Bay to mount a series of IPE pilot projects over a two-year period. The educational model combined a clinical placement for health sciences students with a series of IPE experiences (e.g., weekly tutorials combined with community visits and/or resource sessions). The learning objectives focused on gaining knowledge of the roles of various health professionals and interprofessional collaboration in the context of northern health care. Project evaluation included quantitative and qualitative measures. Outcomes of interest included learner satisfaction, changes in student perceptions, and acquisition of knowledge. Student participation was voluntary and no formal assessment or grading of student performance was required.

Students from the occupational therapy, physiotherapy, medicine, nursing, and midwifery programs at McMaster University who were assigned to clinical placements in Northern Ontario were invited to participate. Students were selected and grouped on the basis of placement dates and geographic location (Thunder Bay, Kenora, or Sioux Lookout) to ensure a critical mass and interprofessional mix of learners. A co-tutor model using individuals from different health professions was used to role model interprofessional collaboration and to expand the interprofessional mix within each group. Tutors were drawn from the pool of clinical faculty and community clinicians.

While IPE experiences were organized around McMaster students, students on placement from other colleges and universities were invited to attend. The purpose of tutorial sessions was for students to discuss each other's roles and the potential for collaboration in the management of actual patients/clients they had encountered during their clinical placements. Paper problems depicting common clinical scenarios were provided to tutors for discussion purposes. There were opportunities for additional learning experiences including resource sessions, community visits, and shadowing other health professionals.

Quantitative and qualitative measures were used to evaluate the learning processes and outcomes. Students completed the Interprofessional Education Perception Scale (Leucht et al. 1990) pre- and post-experience to determine if any changes in their perceptions occurred during the project. Students were also encouraged to keep a weekly journal to document and reflect on their learning experiences prior to, during, and immediately following the project. Following the project, students completed a project evaluation form which provided a self-report of learning outcomes, feedback on the learning process, and an overall rating of the learning experience. To complete the project evaluation, feedback was obtained from tutors and preceptors throughout the two-year study.

A total of 136 students from nine universities and four community colleges participated in 13 pilot projects over the two-year period. There were no differences between participants' pre-test and post-test scores on the Interprofessional Education Perception Scale suggesting that no change in perception had occurred as a result of the IPE experience. A difference between professions was observed in that both physiotherapy and occupational therapy students had more positive perceptions of interprofessional collaboration than did medical students.

Of the 46 students who completed project evaluation forms, 95 percent rated the overall learning experience as 7 (good) or higher on a 10-point scale with 20 percent rating it as 10 (excellent). All of the respondents reported they would recommend this experience to fellow students.

Thirty-five students submitted journals related to their IPE learning experience. Four common themes emerged during the qualitative analysis which indicated students gained new knowledge and insights into: (1) the roles of other health professionals and the potential for interprofessional collaboration, (2) the process of interprofessional learning, (3) aboriginal culture, spirituality, and health beliefs, and (4) health system issues related to access and service delivery in rural and remote regions. Some quotes to illustrate the first two "interprofessional" themes are provided below.

Roles of Health Professionals and Interprofessional Collaboration

It was clear that students gained new knowledge related to each other's roles and how they could work together as a team in the provision of health care. Although most students were familiar with the scope of practice of medicine, nursing, and physiotherapy, many gained new knowledge about other professions such as midwifery, pharmacy, social work, and occupational therapy.

» I was able to have a somewhat better understanding of what some of the other professions do and how we can work together. (Physiotherapy student)

I really enjoyed the opportunity to meet and listen to other tutorial group members, specifically the student social worker and the student midwife. (Medical student)

Process of Interprofessional Learning

Students identified both enablers and barriers to the learning process. Although the majority of students agreed on the benefits of informal learning in social situations, their feedback was inconsistent with regards to the format and structure of the tutorial sessions. For example, some students really enjoyed community outings and resource sessions with native elders while others would have preferred spending more time in tutorial sessions discussing real patients and each other's roles. Similarly, some enjoyed the lack of structure (no formal weekly objectives, no "homework" or formal presentations) while others wanted more structure and/or tutor guidance.

>> I appreciated the supportive, unstructured nature of the group and the facilitators were excellent. (Social Work student)

This tutorial combined with the living arrangements with someone from another profession as well as the social opportunities furthered the education. (Occupational Therapy student)

Tutors agreed that more learning occurred in groups with a broader interprofessional mix of students. The use of a co-tutor model with tutors of different backgrounds also served to expand the interprofessional mix. Tutors agreed that frequent changes in group membership (as students rotated in and out of clinical placements) had a negative impact on group process. While some tutors, like some students, suggested the need for more structure such as formalized weekly case presentations and a mandated shadowing experience for each student, other tutors preferred the informal nature of the tutorial discussions and the increased autonomy provided to students. Regardless of tutor style, all tutors appreciated having a bank of paper problems to use for case discussion if students did not bring their own client cases or issues forward.

In summary, it was clear that most students enjoyed their interprofessional learning experience and would recommend it to others. Although the 13 projects were guided by a similar educational model, student learning experiences varied significantly, depending on student interests, tutor style, and community setting/resources. The importance of such a flexible and student-driven curriculum was reaffirmed; however, feedback suggests the need for some structure and more tutor guidance in order to help students meet individual and group learning objectives. The level of learner (junior versus senior) did not appear to have a negative impact on the learning experience.

Although the pilot phase of this project was completed in December 2002, the Ministry of Health continues to fund this initiative and an additional 100 students have participated in a variety of IPE experiences during their clinical placements in Northern Ontario. The three communities and pool of faculty tutors have remained committed to IPE and plans are being developed to expand IPE into other communities.

In 2002, another new IPE initiative was implemented related to rehabilitation issues in HIV. The complexity of HIV/AIDS from social, psychological, biological, and ethical perspectives was thought to be ideally suited to an interprofessional educational approach. While a few IPE initiatives in relation to HIV have been described, these did not appear to promote the understanding of the roles of other health professionals (Strauss et al. 1992) and have limited the number of professional groups participating in the program of study (Bagolun et al. 1998). The following example describes a problem-based tutorial course related to HIV and rehabilitation that includes five professional groups (Solomon et al. 2003b). One of the core objectives of the course was to increase the understanding of the roles of other health professionals in a rehabilitation model of HIV management.

Senior-level student volunteers from the occupational therapy, physiotherapy, medicine, nursing, and social work programs were invited to participate in an eight-week interprofessional tutorial course entitled "Rehabilitation Issues in HIV". Those interested were invited to submit a brief letter outlining why they were interested in the project and their commitment to attend. Students were selected based on their seniority, motivation, willingness to attend all sessions, and insight into the complexities of HIV/AIDS. Two students from each of the programs were selected from the applicants to form two tutorial groups of five students.

The groups were co-facilitated by a faculty tutor and a person living with HIV who assumed the role of a "resource tutor." The role of the resource tutor was to provide insight from the clients' perspective and prompt and question students to consider varying aspects of the problem (Solomon et al. 2003a). The two-hour tutorial sessions were held weekly over an eight-week period.

Students kept a journal describing and reflecting upon their experiences in the tutorial. They were asked to reflect on their personal objectives, any challenges and successes they encountered in the tutorial setting, personal learning that occurred as a result of participating in the project, and any other general perceptions about their experiences. At the completion of the project, all students, tutors, and resource tutors participated in a semi-structured interview. All interviews were audiotaped and transcribed verbatim.

Nine of ten students completed the course; one medical student was unable to free herself from clinical responsibilities after four weeks of participation. A qualitative content analysis resulted in the identification of a number of themes and subthemes that reflected the students' experiences and perceptions.

■ **1. Factual Knowledge.** Not surprisingly students referred to discussion and learning within the tutorial setting that was related to knowledge and facts about the natural history, the pathology, and related signs of symptoms of HIV/AIDS. The students also gained increased knowledge and understanding of the roles of the other disciplines. Students developed awareness of their preconceived stereotypes of other professions and appeared to gain a greater respect and appreciation of the contributions of others.

>> I have also begun to understand what each profession brings to the care of the patient. It has been extremely beneficial because each one has certain knowledge and approaches to situations. I have appreciated the variety of assessment tools and resource information that they bring to class. (journal – Occupational Therapy)

Before this class I had strong opinions, which were based on prior experience with Dr.'s. When I met the med student, she changed that for me. It is important to study and work together so we are not separate silos operating under different parts of a system. (journal – Social Work).

■ **2. Benefits of Interprofessional Learning.** There were many journal entries and interview references related to the benefits of the interprofessional design of the course. Students developed an increased awareness of how much more they achieved when they worked together and of how they were able to build on each other's knowledge to increase their learning.

>> I think the biggest thing was that how much knowledge…how much everyone in the team can learn from each other. I think it was demonstrated every single week. And we brought in stuff and realized that everyone is able to fill the gaps of everyone else – and if we could rely on each other more as a team than just as individual health care providers the amount of good you can do for someone just multiplies itself. (interview – Nursing)

Students wrote of the increased breadth of learning that occurred from interacting with students from other disciplines.

>> I especially appreciate the perspectives from social work, the PT and the OT…the nurses too, but their roles are similar to mine, or at least their approaches seem to be. (journal – Medicine)

■ **3. Rehabilitation Insight.** Students seemed to gain a broader understanding of rehabilitation and insight into the importance of client-centered practice in a rehabilitation model of practice. They developed an appreciation that different professions had slightly different interpretations of rehabilitation.

>> I never knew that there were so many ways and means to energy conserve for example. And just with someone who's very fatigued and may not have the energy reserves that they need to do their daily activities – I had no idea. Like that you could have special spoons and special carts that allow you to transport food and all these kind of things that we never discuss in my particular profession. (interview – Medicine)

A sense of confidence in knowing their profession-specific role in dealing with someone with HIV/AIDS also emerged in the analysis of the journals. Through explaining and advocating for their disciplinary role the students also learned more about what their specific profession could offer and of the applicability of their knowledge and skills.

>> …not a lot of us had a lot of experience with [HIV] but you can rely on so many other things you've learned in your past and apply it to so many different situations and things that we hadn't really thought about that we could do for someone with HIV that you are doing for other clients too. (interview – Nursing)

■ **4. Enjoyment.** Although this experience was in addition to their regular academic and clinical studies, students reflected on a sense of enjoyment. They described how their tutorial experience changed their thinking and provided insights. Some of the enjoyment stemmed from the fact that this was an interprofessional learning experience.

>> I am learning so much from the members of my tutorials, their different professions and their roles with people living with HIV. I am very eager to begin the next case scenario next week. (journal – Occupational Therapy)

For the first time I am seeing and feeling the breadth of health care. It's great…I really feel like my understanding of health care is opening up. (journal – Medicine)

This course provides an example of a successful small group problem-based IPE experience which was disease-specific. The topic area of HIV and rehabilitation was ideal for learning and discussion around the values, skills, and knowledge of the professions. Others have described incorporating small group discussions into their HIV educational initiatives. It was our experience that the eight-week duration of the course was an important component of the design as it allowed the students to develop longer term relationships and for a high level of honesty and disclosure that would be difficult to achieve in a single session.

Summary/Lessons Learned

Many of the challenges we encountered in our attempts to integrate IPE into the occupational therapy and physiotherapy curricula over the years have been reported by others. Some issues, however, are probably unique to our educational institution where self-directed learning, problem-based learning, and small group learning are sacrosanct pedagogical principles. Nonetheless, many lessons have been learned along the way in our IPE journey that may be of interest to others. These lessons are discussed below from the perspective of the educational institution, the faculty/curriculum planners, and the students.

From the Institutional Perspective

The most critical factor for the success of IPE is the need to establish a new IPE culture within the educational institution. Ideally, IPE should be captured in the mission statement and/or expressed values of the organization. As the literature suggests, "rigid academic hierarchies" (Erickson et al. 1998 p. 147) must be broken down, and the silo approach to the education of health professionals must be replaced with more collaborative models (Bainbridge and Matthews 1996; Cleary and Howell 2003) so that faculty from various professional backgrounds and disciplines are truly encouraged and supported to work together to develop and deliver the IPE curriculum. Stumpf and Clark (1999 p. 31) have discussed "burying the hatchet", "status protection," and "identity protectionism" as barriers to IPE. Faculty who can collaborate to deliver IPE become important role models for both faculty colleagues and students. Dedicated and committed faculty, including champions for specific IPE events or courses, become key ingredients to make IPE both viable in the short term and sustainable in the long term. While we have many faculty who are committed to IPE and have devoted time and energy to IPE in addition to their regular workload, we have learned that it is important that all faculty get "credit" for IPE teaching as part of their overall responsibilities.

An institutional policy to support mandatory versus optional IPE would serve not only to facilitate faculty buy-in but also to stress the importance of IPE to students (Banks and Janke 1998; Erickson et al. 1998; Pringle et al. 2000). Without an integrated IPE core curriculum, student workload is increased since students must choose to attend optional IPE events. This problem has been discussed by others (Erikson et al. 1998; Richardson et al. 1997; Tryssenaar et al. 1996).

Costs related to IPE are significant (Cloonan et al. 1999; Erikson et al. 1998; Erkel et al. 1995). Internal funding in terms of a base budget allocation is necessary to support IPE in terms of long-term sustainability since external funding for pilot projects is short-lived. Finally, a change of organizational structure to support a new trans-professional IPE division, department, or program, headed by a faculty member with a recognized portfolio and leadership skills along with a group of dedicated faculty members, would provide a clear message to all stakeholders regarding the importance of IPE within the educational institution. In summary, for IPE to be successful, institutional commitment is needed in terms of organizational culture, mission statement, structure, funding, educational policy, and dedicated faculty role models.

From the Faculty/Curriculum Planning Perspective

Based on our experience, the biggest and most pragmatic barrier for faculty planners to overcome in implementing IPE is student timetable conflicts. Others have discussed the difficulty in gaining faculty cooperation to change student schedules in order to introduce IPE into the curriculum (Harden 1998; Larson 1995; Stumpf and Clark 1999; Yarborough et al. 2000). Freeman et al. (2000) point to professional differences in our basic values and philosophies of teamwork as contributing factors to this problem. Our experience suggests that the medical faculty and students are the most difficult group to convince regarding the importance of IPE. Although Schmitt (2001) agrees that medicine has little interest in interprofessional activities, Barr (2001 p. 20) states: "suggestions that doctors and medical students are reluctant joiners are not bourn out by the facts."

It is very clear to us that isolated one-day events are not only resource-intensive but also limited in terms of effectiveness. Students reported greater satisfaction and improved learning outcomes with longer exposure to IPE interventions. A similar dose-response relationship was reported by Mu et al. (2004); however, the evidence regarding the ideal length of exposure to IPE remains unclear.

Our experience also suggests that IPE can be effective in both classroom and clinical settings. While the clinical settings would appear to provide a more applied and realistic venue, we have learned that it is important to include clinical and community partners early in the planning stage to maximize buy-in and diffuse issues related to power control. It is also clear that student learning is maximized with a greater mix of professions, when student interaction and teamwork is required, and when rotating group membership is minimized.

Although IPE can be effective in the context of a specific topic or patient population, such as ethics, HIV/AIDS, or native health issues, it is important that the IPE intervention focus on understanding the roles of other health professionals and the benefits of team decision making. This required faculty to clearly delineate learning objectives, expectations of students, and evaluation requirements. For example, if using paper or simulated patient problems for IPE, they must be designed carefully to generate the desired learning issues that focus on professional roles and collaboration versus the underlying bio-psycho-social issues which students are typically used to exploring. In other words, the disease-specific and profession-specific content should be minimized and the interprofessional content maximized.

Our experience also suggests that students at any level can benefit from IPE; however, the evidence supporting this notion remains unclear (Byrne 1991; Harden 1998; van der Horst et al. 1995). On the one hand, there is a perceived need for students to develop their own professional identity including "awareness of their profession's values, traditions, aims and goals" (Byrne 1991 p. 3) before engaging in IPE activities. On the other hand, it can be argued that early introduction of IPE is required to prevent entrenchment in one's profession. Regardless of when IPE is introduced, the context of the learning experience must fit with program or course objectives so that students are motivated to learn. Similarly, IPE experiences should include a student evaluation component since this drives student learning and confirms the importance of the learning for the student.

Finally, we have learned that informal learning is important and perhaps more significant than originally expected. Students can learn to trust one another and acquire new knowledge related to IPE while they are socializing, playing, and living together. The formal classroom activities can thus act as a catalyst to foster informal learning opportunities where additional learning occurs or at least is reinforced.

From the Student Perspective

It is clear from our experience and the literature that students enjoy IPE when it involves sharing ideas, debating options, problem-solving, and reaching shared decisions. Students learn about each other's roles and appreciate the need for collaboration. Some students gain confidence in their own role and the unique expertise they have to contribute to the team. When IPE is offered as an optional experience, some students perceive it as an interesting but unnecessary "add-on" to their already busy schedule and they resent giving up their profession-specific learning activities (Johnson 2003).

Although we have learned much about IPE, several questions remain unanswered and require further study: (1) the ideal dose/duration of IPE required to make a difference in attitudes and practice behaviors of future health professionals, (2) the ideal level of learner (junior versus senior) and timing of introduction into the curriculum to optimize the impact of IPE, and (3) the ideal IPE instructor/tutor in terms of interests, values, skills, and professional development needs.

Many obstacles exist to implementing IPE activities; however, the need to overcome them is critical if we are to keep pace with the changing health care system and better prepare health professional students for collaborative practice. We have experienced many failures but have also enjoyed many successes over the last twenty years in our attempts to integrate IPE in the occupational therapy and physiotherapy programs at McMaster. We look forward to the future with renewed enthusiasm and wisdom having learned from our mistakes!

A Glimpse at the Future of Interprofessional Education at McMaster University

A new IPE Working Group has been established in the Faculty of Health Sciences with a mandate to develop an IPE curriculum for all health sciences students. While our Canadian colleagues at the University of British Columbia (Gilbert et al. 2000) and the University of Alberta (Taylor et al. 2004) have chosen to mount a required course for all health professional students, we have decided to pursue an educational model that is more consistent with our philosophy of problem-based, self-directed, small group learning. We envision a menu of IPE offerings in which students will participate (based on their personal learning needs and learning style) to accumulate a required number of credits/hours over the course of their professional training. The menu will focus on active and interactive learning and will include a variety of IPE activities that vary in terms of format, duration, and location, and include activities such as communication skills laboratories/workshops, team placements, group projects, ePBL/online tutorials, shadowing experiences, and lectures/seminars.

The list of collaborative competencies outlined by Barr (2001) will serve to guide the process of curriculum development:

- Describe one's roles and responsibilities clearly to other professions and discharge them to the satisfaction of those others

- Recognize and observe the constraints of one's role, responsibilities and competence yet perceive needs in a wider context

- Recognize and respect the roles, responsibilities and competence of other professions in relation to one's own, knowing when, where and how to involve others through agreed channels

- Work with other professions to review services, effect change, improve standards, solve problems and resolve conflict in the provision of care and treatment

- Work with other professions to assess, plan, provide and review care for individual patients and support careers

- Tolerate differences, misunderstandings, ambiguities, shortcomings and unilateral change in another profession

- Enter into interdependent relationships, teaching and sustaining other professions and learning from and being sustained by those other professions

- Facilitate interprofessional case conferences, meetings, team working and networking

A framework adapted from Hammick (2000) will serve to guide the evaluation process. Potential outcomes of interest include: learner reaction/satisfaction, changes in attitudes/perceptions, changes in knowledge, changes in skills, changes in practice behavior, changes in organizational culture and structure, and improved health outcomes. The first four are deemed to be appropriate for evaluating student learning in the short term but the final three outcomes will require long-term follow-up studies.

The next steps in the curriculum development process include seeking approval from the various Program Education Committees to support a mandatory IPE core curriculum, recruiting faculty, piloting several new initiatives, soliciting feedback from all stakeholder groups, establishing an administrative structure for IPE activities and resources, and securing funding support. A mammoth task but one we are committed to following through!

References

Bainbridge L, Matthews ML (1996) Towards new strategies for managing change in the health professions: a joint initiative. Health Management Resources Group, Vancouver, BC

Balogun J, Kaplan M, Miller T (1998) The effect of professional education on the knowledge and attitudes of physical therapist and occupational therapist students about acquired immunodeficiency syndrome. Phys Ther 79: 1073–1082

Banks S, Janke K (1998) Developing and implementing interprofessional learning in a faculty of health professions. J Allied Health 27: 132–136

Barr H (2001) Interprofessional education: today, yesterday and tomorrow. Learning and Teaching Support Network Centre of Health Sciences and Practice, Westminster University, London, UK

Barr H, Hammick M, Koppel I, Reeves S (1999) Systematic review of the effectiveness of interprofessional education: towards transatlantic collaboration. J Allied Health 28:104–108

Byrne C (1991) Interdisciplinary education in undergraduate health sciences. Pedagogue (Perspectives on Health Sciences Education, published by McMaster University, Faculty of Health Sciences) 3:1–8

Clark PG (1997) Values in health care professional socialization: implications for geriatric education in interdisciplinary teamwork. Gerontologist 37:441–451

Cleary KK, Howell DM (2003) The educational interaction between physical therapy and occupational therapy students. J Allied Health 32:71–77

Cloonan PA, Davis FD, Burnett CB (1999) Interdisciplinary education in clinical ethics: a work in progress. Holist Nurs Pract 13:12–19

Cooper H, Carlisle C, Gibbs T, Watkins C (2001) Developing an evidence base for interdisciplinary learning: a systematic review. J Adv Nurs 35:228–237

Erickson B, McHarney-Brown C, Seeger K, Kaufman A (1998) Overcoming barriers to interprofessional health sciences education. Educ Health 11:143–149

Erkel EA, Nivens AS, Kennedy DE (1995) Intensive immersion of nursing students in rural interdisciplinary care. J Nurs Educ 34:359–365

Freeman M, Miller C, Ross N (2000) The impact of individual philosophies of teamwork on multi-professional practice and the implications for education. J Interprof Care 14:237–246

Freeth D, Hammick M, Koppel I, Reeves S, Barr H (2002) A critical review of evaluations of interprofessional education, discussion paper no. 2. Centre for Health Sciences and Practice, London, UK

Gilbert JHV, Camp RD, Cole CD, Bruce C, Fieldings DW, Stanton SJ (2000) Preparing students for interprofessional teamwork in health care. J Interprof Care 14:223–234

Hammick M (2000) Interprofessional education: evidence from the past to guide the future. Med Teach 22:461–467

Harden RM (1998) MMEE guide no. 12: multiprofessional education, part 1. Effective multiprofessional education: a three-dimensional perspective. Med Teach 20:402–408

Irvine R, Kerridge I, McPhee J, Freeman S (2002) Interprofessionalism and ethics: consensus or clash of cultures? J Interprof Care 16:199–210

Johnson R (2003) Exploring students' views of interprofessional education. Int J Ther Rehabil 10:314–320

Larson EL (1995) New rules for the game: interdisciplinary education. Nurs Outlook 43:180–185

Leucht RM, Madsen MK, Taugher MP, Petterson BJ (1990) Assessing professional perceptions: design and validation of an interdisciplinary education perception scale. J Allied Health 19:181–191

Mu K, Chao CC, Jensen GM, Royeen CB (2004) Effects of interprofessional rural training on students' perceptions of interprofessional health care services. J Allied Health 33:125–131

Pringle D, Levitt C, Horsburgh M, Wilson R, Whittaker M (2000) Interdisciplinary collaboration and primary heath care reform. Can Fam Physician 46:763–765

Richardson J, Montemuro M, Cripps D, Mohide EA, Macpherson AS (1997) Educating students for interprofessional teamwork in the clinical placement setting. Educ Gerontol 23:669–693

Richardson J, Montemuro M, Mohide EA, Cripps D, Macpherson AS (1999) Training for interprofessional teamwork: evaluation of an undergraduate experience. Educ Gerontol 25:411–434

Romanow R (2002) Building on values: the future of health care in Canada. National Library of Canada, Ottawa, ON

Schmitt M (2001) Collaboration improves the quality of care: methodological challenges and evidence from US health care research. J Interprof Care 15:2–21

Singleton JK, Green-Hernandez C (1998) Interdisciplinary education and practice: has its time come? J Nurse Midwifery 43:3–7

Solomon P, Guenter D, Salvatori P (2003a) Integration of persons with HIV in a problem-based tutorial: a qualitative study. Teach Learn Med 15:257–261

Solomon P, Salvatori P, Guenter D (2003b) An interprofessional problem-based learning course on rehabilitation issues in HIV. Med Teach 25:408–413

Strauss R, Corless I, Luckey J, van der Horst C, Dennis B (1992) Cognitive and attitudinal impacts of a university AIDS course: interdisciplinary education as a public health intervention. Am J Public Health 82:569–572

Stumpf SH, Clark JZ (1999) The promise and pragmatism of interdisciplinary education. J Allied Health 28:30–32

Taylor E, Cook D, Cunningham R, King S, Pimlott J (2004) Changing attitudes: health sciences students working together. Internet J Allied Health Sci Pract 2:1–13

Tryssenaar J, Perkins J, Brett L (1996) Undergraduate interdisciplinary education: are we educating for future practice? Can J Occup Ther 63:245–251

Van der Horst M, Turpie I, Nelson W, Cole B, Sammon S, Sniderman P, Tremblay M (1995) St. Joseph's Community Health Centre model of community-based interdisciplinary health care team education. Health Soc Care Community 3:33–42

World Health Organization (1978) Learning together to work together for health. WHO, Geneva (technical report series 769)

Yarborough M, Jones T, Cyr T, Phillips S, Stelzner D (2000) Interprofessional education in ethics at an academic health sciences center. Acad Med 75:793–800

Zwarenstein M, Reeves S, Barr H, Hammick M, Kippel I, Atkins J (2002) Interprofessional education: effects on professional practice and health care outcomes (Cochrane Review). The Cochrane Library, Issue 4, Update Software, Oxford

Chapter 8

Curricula to Promote Community Health

Julie Richardson, Lori Letts

Contents

This chapter outlines the curricula in community health and community practice in the Physiotherapy and Occupational Therapy Programs at McMaster University. The two programs have taken different approaches to incorporating community content. In the Physiotherapy Program, the development of this curriculum was a major shift reflecting a change of practice from acute to ambulatory settings and an emerging expansion of the professional role. Occupational therapy practice has historically been grounded within everyday occupations within the community. The occupational therapy curriculum is integrated throughout the two-year curriculum, while in Physiotherapy it is concentrated in a Community Health/Community Practice Unit. For this reason, to provide the most clarity, descriptions of the curricula in the two programs are presented separately. While there are similarities in issues across the curricula, for example in the models of practice through consultation and mediation, there are differences in how these are structured.

Community Health/Community Practice in the Physiotherapy Program

Impetus for Change

The delivery of health care has changed dramatically in the past 10–15 years, with a greater emphasis on ambulatory care and an increase in the acuity of patients seen in the hospital, outpatient, and home care settings. In response to this change academic programs must prepare physiotherapists with a different set of skills that emphasize community health education and disease prevention. Traditionally physiotherapy interventions have been primarily focused toward tertiary interventions that aim to halt the secondary effect or disability associated with a disease. This new approach refocuses interventions toward primary and secondary prevention. Primary prevention addresses the prevention of the disease itself while secondary prevention involves targeting persons who have risk factors for the disease and associated preclinical disease (Fletcher et al. 1982).

Another impetus for redirecting the curriculum is the changing demographic profile of the population. From 1979 to 2000, life expectancy for men increased by 5.4 years and for women by 3.2 years (Statistics Canada 2002). In 1996, at birth, Canadian men could expect to live 66.9 years without disability while women would spend 70.2 years in this state. In the same year, at 65 years the expected years of disability-free life for men were 10.9 and 12.4 for women (Statistics Canada 2002). This shift in demographics has been accompanied by a corresponding increase in the prevalence of chronic disease.

The ideal healthy population would have long life expectancy with the effects of chronic disease compressed into a very short time before death (Fries 1987). Epidemiological transition theories explain large-scale changes in population indicators, mortality, and morbidity. There is currently a resurgence of infectious diseases along with a major transition from acute to chronic, degenerative diseases such as heart disease, cerebrovascular disease, type II diabetes, and chronic obstructive respiratory disease (Olshansky and Ault 1986; Omran 1971; Rogers and Hackenberg 1987). If there is an increase in the prevalence of diseases that have a high rate of mobility problems and associated physical disability (e.g., osteoarthritis, diabetes), the prevalence of disability within the general population will also increase (Adams and Wilkins 1992; Colvez and Blanchett 1983; Manton 1988; van de Water and Perenboom 1996).

This will increase the number of persons who could potentially benefit from expertise offered by physiotherapists.

Canadians will spend the last 10 years of their life, on average, being limited in at least one activity, and thus classified as having a disability (Statistics Canada 2002). One major goal of health planners and health care providers is to increase the disability-free life expectancy by delaying the onset of disability. To attain this goal, self-monitoring and/or monitoring of functional health of older adults by health care providers is essential (Gill et al. 2002). Since physiotherapists are movement specialists they have a major role to play in the prevention of the onset of disability.

Globalization continues to have a major impact on health. This is a result of an increased interrelatedness of economies, and an increased movement of people across borders, influencing how individuals and populations interact with each other. The development and use of technology has sped up the spread and control of disease. Technology such as transportation has meant that diseases move quickly throughout the world and information about containment is shared between countries. As well there has been an increase in "cognitive globalization" as a result of advertising and marketing of Western ideals and goods that has led to the spread of lifestyle diseases (Lee 2004; Patrick and Cadman 2002). All these factors will affect how the graduates of today and tomorrow practice and perform within health care teams.

The goal of educational programs in physiotherapy is to prepare clinicians for current and future practice. Various documents have been compiled which emphasize physiotherapists' roles in wellness, health promotion, and disease prevention (American Physical Therapy Association 1997a, b; Commission on Accreditation in Physical Therapy Education 1998). Several documents have been developed to drive curriculum which advance that physiotherapists promote optimal health by providing information on wellness, disease, impairments, functional limitations, disability, and health risks related to age, gender, culture, and lifestyle (American Physical Therapy Association 1997a, b; Commission on Accreditation in Physical Therapy Education 1998). Graduates of physiotherapy programs should have the ability to educate patients or clients on health promotion and on wellness, incorporating the concepts of self-responsibility. They should have the ability to function as consultants in various health care settings and to assess the effectiveness of health promotion and wellness programs. Professional organizations have called for curricula to cover both prevention and wellness programs as they relate to physiotherapy (American Physical Therapy Association 1997b). The American Physical Therapy Association's (1997a) *Guide to Physical Therapy Practice* states that physiotherapists are involved in wellness initiatives including health promotion and education that stimulate the public to engage in healthy behaviors and provide preventive care that forestalls or prevents functional decline and the need for more intense care. As part of the Essential Competencies Profile compiled by academic and professional regulating bodies in Canada, one of three key roles outlined cites that physiotherapists practice along a continuum from primary to tertiary care and focus on educating patients, clients, and others to promote health, wellness, fitness, and self-management (Accreditation Council for Canadian Academic Programs, Canadian Alliance of Physiotherapy Regulators, Canada Physiotherapy Association, and Canadian Universities Physical Therapy Academic Committee 2004). The direction projected for the profession recognizes the contribution we have to make to health care with respect to patient education, promoting healthy lifestyles, and being partners with patients in managing their disease.

Assessment, Communication, and Management of Risk

The objective of the physiotherapy intervention is to improve or maintain the health status of the client or population, primarily through optimizing functional status. Physiotherapists assess the risk factors and protective factors for functional decline that increase or decrease the probability of a certain outcome. Physiotherapists also provide interventions which reduce the level of risk to which an individual or population is exposed. The risk profile of the person should be the focus of any intervention (Martin and Fell 1999). Using measurement tools that have established sensitivity and specificity estimates for the risk factor of interest is essential (Chiu et al. 2003; Riddle and Stratford 1999). Communicating risk to either the individual or another health care provider is not straightforward and requires an understanding of the other person's perspective to effectively communicate your findings. We have had experience with communicating the results of functional assessments through a Functional Status Laboratory that offers annual assessments to community dwelling older adults. The participants receive a verbal report explaining the results of the assessment, and written recommendations about what they could do to improve. Communication of the results to their physician is through a standardized form that conveys the results in a format similar to that of a laboratory result. The results of tests are listed along with sex- and aged-based norms and highlight when the patient falls outside the range for a specific impairment or function. Development of skills and strategies to communicate risk require more attention if physiotherapists are to develop practice in primary and secondary prevention strategies.

Physiotherapists may have input around risk when the management is related to education about a risk factor such as muscle strength and when the intervention will involve more direct management. Muscle strength and balance have been identified as risk factors for falling (Moreland et al. 2003); changes within the environment or personal behaviors may be targeted as part of the risk management strategy to reduce the risk of falling. Physiotherapists may develop health maintenance schedules which offer a method of monitoring patients in primary care at defined intervals depending on their age, gender, and risk factors for primary and/or secondary prevention (Frame 1996).

Physiotherapy Role as Educators of Health Promotion and Disease Prevention

Physiotherapy educators have not exploited health promotion as they develop curriculum and explore the development of professional skills (Gahimer and Morris 1999). The process of enabling people to increase control over, and improve their health through health education, economic, environmental, and organizational supports directed at individuals, groups, and communities needs to be developed within physiotherapy curricula (Green and Anderson 1986; World Health Organization 1986). The issues of disease prevention (i.e., the control of risk factors, the early detection and treatment of disease to prevent deterioration and complications from occurring when disease or disability are already established) have not been well developed or conceptualized for students (Fletcher et al. 1982).

While physiotherapists have always been involved in patient education, this role has expanded to include planned, organized learning experiences designed to facilitate

Resource Sessions

The first resource session prepares students for the different approach in the unit. Prior to the session students are asked to read two papers to prepare and orientate them to the broad issues of health and set the scene for the unit (Last 1998; Minkler 1999). The content of Minkler's paper is crucial to the development of this curriculum. It initiates a paradigm shift from acute care mediated by the health professional to chronic health conditions in which the care is a partnership between the patient and health professional. Minkler discusses the continuing controversies of personal versus social responsibility for health and the positive and negative consequences of an individual being held accountable for his/her own health behavior. The paper makes a case for broader ecological approaches to health that includes individual responsibility within the wider social responsibility. Last (1998) provides an epidemiological perspective about the social and behavioral determinants of health. The introduction to the unit is crucial in providing a framework for the orientation of these new ideas and showing how they relate to physiotherapy practice.

The introductory session follows up on these readings. Students engage in what is called a "health exercise" by asking them to reflect upon their personal definition of health. The outline for this exercise can be seen in Table 8.1. During this session students review the LaLonde report (1974) in which Canada became the first national government to articulate the importance of factors beyond the health care system that promote or diminish health (human biology, environment, lifestyle, and health care organization) (LaLonde 1974). As well students examine the twelve determinants of health that Health Canada recognizes today (Health Canada 2002). After the health exercise we review the definition of community health and the three major functions of public health that have been compiled by the Institute of Medicine (1988) (see Table 8.2). These explanations are described in a way that is particularly relevant to phys-

Table 8.1. Health exercise

What is your definition of health?
What does it mean as you relate it to your own health?
What are your positive health behaviors?
What are your less positive health behaviors?
What do you do to maintain a positive health state within various systems and which system is most important to you?
What other risk or protective factors do you consider important to your own health?
How do considerations of these risks alter your behavior?
Then focusing on one type of health behavior, i.e., physical activity and exercise. How active are you now? How active do you want to be when you are fifty and then seventy? What do you need to do to plan for this?
What are the barriers to your positive health behaviors – what makes you fall off the rails – stops you from maintaining an optimal level of health?
Think of a client in an outpatient setting with whom you were taking a history and became aware that their health behaviors could be improved. What did you do?
How do think that your reaction as a health practitioner has been impacted by your values, beliefs, and knowledge?

Table 8.2. Community and public health definitions

What is community health?	Three major functions of public health
The science and art of preventing disease, prolonging life, and promoting health and efficiency through organized community effort (Institute of Medicine 1988)	Assessment: assessing and monitoring the health of communities and populations at risk to identify health problems and priorities
	Policy development: formulating public policies in collaboration with community and government leaders designed to solve identified local and national health problems and priorities
	Assurance: assuring that all populations have access to appropriate and cost-effective care, including health promotion and disease prevention services, and evaluation of the effectiveness of that care (Institute of Medicine 1988)

iotherapy making the obvious link between musculoskeletal health and practitioners who are experts in this field. Finally students are asked to recall a clinical interaction when they addressed a health issue/behavior with a patient that was not the prime reason for referral.

Another resource session focuses on the role of physiotherapy in global health initiatives. A faculty member of a community health network discusses the role of the physiotherapist in global health. He/she presents the results of a SWOT Analysis (S = Strengths, W = Weakness, O = Opportunities and T = Threats) examining the potential role of the physiotherapy in future global health initiatives and describes his/her experience in developing countries (Landry et al. (2002). Several students chose to do their final clinical placement overseas in a third world country and this session helps them to examine issues involved in delivering rehabilitation services in this context.

Evaluation Methods

A variety of evaluation methods reflect the different focus of the unit. Students are required to keep a journal outlining their preconceptions prior to the unit and reflecting on the material they encounter during the unit. They are also required to write two papers. In the first paper students develop a new, or not commonly used, model of physiotherapy practice using a theory introduced in the unit. The second paper requires students to select and critically appraise a scientific paper that assesses a community-based intervention aimed at modifying an outcome(s) that is associated with multiple risk factors. Students develop a scenario that reflects a public health issue within a community, such as falls in older adults, and then search for a paper that addresses this issue (Tinnetti et al. (1994).

The final evaluation is a group project where students develop an educational package that is client-centered, self-paced, and promotes empowerment of clients in the management of their conditions. Students use all types of media such as web sites, video-discs, brochures, and workbooks in the development of this package.

Challenges with this Curriculum

There have been many challenges in the development of this curriculum. The first is that profession-specific literature to support many of the concepts is sparse and students often use literature generated by other disciplines to explore their learning issues. The physiotherapy roles created within the problems in the tutorial course are emerging roles and therefore examples of these roles for students are limited. Clinical faculty recruited to this unit, as tutors, are physiotherapists who are interested in community roles and issues. However, much of the curriculum is related to roles that are not mainstream and so there is new learning for tutors and students alike. The information disseminated at workshops, tutors' meeting, and resources about the content need to be more comprehensive than in those in other units where knowledge is assumed.

An additional challenge relates to the fact that not all students identify with, or put a high priority on, their role as a health educator. Some students are more interested in acute illness rather than chronic disease and issues of self-management, and do not see the relevance of the material. This attitude often changes after recent graduates attend the class and share their views on how useful they found many of the skills and concepts of the unit.

Future Development and Research

The Community Health/Community Practice unit in the physiotherapy program described in this chapter has been part of the curriculum for three years and has experienced several iterations. The implementation of this curriculum has been exciting and timely with the changes in health care delivery to community practice and primary care. It has received a positive response from students but is not always totally embraced when the content is not viewed as core to the profession.

There are always areas that require further development and thought especially in an area of practice in which the role for physiotherapists is evolving and emerging. Future development in this curriculum will need to provide a more focused framework for home care practice and to address issues on the relationship between adherence to unsupervised practice of exercise/skills, self-efficacy, and other known mediators. Native and cultural issues as they relate to health need to be more comprehensively addressed (Jensen and Lorish 1994). The integration of physiotherapy into Primary Care settings also needs to be explored in conjunction with educating students about the role of physiotherapy in self-management programs. A brief international survey of the community health curriculum in other programs was completed recently and this information will be used to inform future development of the curriculum.

The McMaster Experience (Occupational Therapy)

In Canadian Occupational Therapy practice, community practice has increased and evolved significantly in recent years. For example in 1999, 17.6 percent of members of the Canadian Association of Occupational Therapists (CAOT) identified the client's home as their primary practice setting. By 2003, this had increased to 20.6 percent (Canadian Association of Occupational Therapists 1999, 2004a, b). Occupational therapists' work in and with communities goes well beyond the home setting. Other community settings include workplaces, schools, and primary care. A number of occupational therapists work as members of community-based teams providing services to adults with mental illness (through assertive community treatment teams, clubhouses, and outreach initiatives), children with disabilities (through school-based and community center-based initiatives), and older adults (through active living programs, primary care settings, and community centers).

A number of position statements from CAOT argue for a need to ensure that occupational therapists are prepared to work to promote community health. For example in 2000, CAOT (2000a) affirmed its position that home care is an essential component of Canada's health care service, and that occupational therapists can contribute effectively to the health of Canadians through this model of service delivery. In the same year, CAOT identified that "occupational therapy has a critical role in primary health care" (CAOT 2000b p. 357) and identified roles in a number of sectors including health, education, housing, employment, environmental design, health promotion and injury prevention, and community development. More recently, there have been position statements on topics related to community practice and community health including active living for older adults (CAOT 2003a), universal design (CAOT 2003b), healthy occupations for children and youth (CAOT 2004a), and workplace health (CAOT 2004b). The trends in practice and position statements provide support for, and are reflective of, occupational therapy practice that has been shifting to the community.

Definitions of Community and Community Health

Various definitions of community can be noted in the community health and community organizing literature. Bulmer (1987) notes that community is a normative as well as an analytic and descriptive concept. As such it is a word that conveys values while also conveying a sense of structure. Common definitions relate to geographic areas or clusters of people with shared characteristics such as interests, religion, occupation, illnesses, or disabilities. After review and analysis of sociological conceptualizations of community, Bulmer concludes that a working definition of community should include identification of locally based informal social networks together with a sense of belonging. Drevdahl (1995) describes two definitions of community that lead to different responses in terms of understanding and addressing community health concerns. She notes that "community is considered either a single entity or a collection of unique individuals" (Drevdahl 1995 p. 14), and that each of those definitions, based on differing ideologies, result in different actions in community to address health concerns. Clearly community is a word that has multiple definitions, and it may be important to be explicit about that definition in the context in which it is used.

Despite the increased emphasis on community in practice, there is no singular accepted definition of community or community health in occupational therapy. Scaffa (2001) in her book on community-based practice of occupational therapy reviews a number of different definitions of community. These definitions include people with shared geography or other interest. Christiansen and Townsend (2004 p. 142) take a slightly different focus by describing human communities as "groups of people who do things together and individually." Similarly, occupational therapy has not adopted a singular definition of community health. Rather a number of models or approaches to service delivery have evolved as increasing numbers of occupational therapists practice in the context of community.

Models of Occupational Therapy in the Community

Many occupational therapists believe that their practice is grounded in the context of community, regardless of its location. For example, occupational therapists working in inpatient settings are always cognizant of the need to consider the home and community setting to which their individual clients will return. However, occupational therapy that is provided in community settings is frequently different in that it is often based in organizations that do not necessarily subscribe to medical models.

For occupational therapists, a distinction can be made in types of community practice. Although these are not often referred to as models of practice, they do represent different approaches or ways to organize community occupational therapy practice. There are instances in which occupational therapy practice is provided "in" the community, while in others it is considered to be practice "with" the community. Often this distinction also reflects the level at which the work is being undertaken. For example, working with individual clients in home, school, or workplace settings may be more likely to reflect practice in the community. Community settings are the site of the practice, with the focus on assisting the individual client in finding ways to engage in optimal occupational performance to meet the demands and expectations of various roles. When practice is with groups of people in community settings, it often involves working in partnership with the group; working with the community group to meet the goals of the group, often by making changes to the community itself. Examples of this in the context of health promotion and community development have been described in the occupational therapy literature (Banks and Head 2004; Letts et al. 1993).

McComas and Carswell (1994) propose a model for community-based health promotion that provides a visual depiction of this idea. Their model incorporates iterative expansions into community contexts, beginning with individual empowerment, and expanding to small group development, community organization, coalition advocacy, and political action. Their model provides a way to organize occupational therapy efforts to promote health at the level of the individual and moving into working in partnership with organizations. Their model also leaves room for diverse approaches to practice to promote health in and with communities. This diversity of approaches is reflected in the occupational therapy program at McMaster University.

Examples from the Occupational Therapy Program

Within McMaster University's occupational therapy curriculum, students are exposed to knowledge, skills, and professional behaviors that will prepare them for practice both in and with the community. In the occupational therapy program, community content is integrated across the entire curriculum. A brief summary highlighting the community content in each term is provided here, with emphasis on particular assignments, clinical scenarios, and instructional sessions that emphasize community practice.

Term 1: Health, Wellness, and Occupation

Since the first term of the program is described in relation to health and wellness, a major focus is gaining an understanding of these terms and how they are used in occupational therapy. In the second week of class, a large group inquiry seminar introduces the students to concepts of health, health promotion, and public health. They are exposed to international documents such as the Ottawa Charter for Health Promotion (World Health Organization [WHO] 1986), and how this model and others have been linked to occupational therapy (Finlayson and Edwards 1997; Thibeault and Hebert 1997). Later in that term, a large group session focuses on global health issues, and a resource session is offered to orient the students to the International Classification of Functioning, Disability and Health (WHO 2001). Problem scenarios in the problem-based tutorials in the first term also provide the students with grounding in community and community health. For example, one scenario follows the same person with Down Syndrome from birth, as he enters kindergarten, and as he completes high school, placing his life experiences within his community context. Another scenario focuses on an occupational therapist providing consultation through a community health center to a recreation program that is working to increase its accessibility.

Within this term, the students are also introduced to perspectives on disability. They are linked with volunteers who have varying types of disabilities and are given an opportunity to "shadow" the volunteer for a minimum of two hours. This experience and the reflective summary that they are required to submit encourage the students to consider the factors within the community that both impede and enhance an individual's participation, and to reflect on the experience of living in the community with a disability.

Term 2: Person, Environment, and Occupation

Term 2 in part places an emphasis on understandings of environments, including community environments. In one inquiry seminar session, students are exposed to theories of person–environment relations. In groups they complete assignments involving review of concepts or theories relevant to community and community health. For example, students examine the underlying principles of either universal design or ergonomics, both of which are important to community-based practice. In their problem-based tutorials, problem scenarios encompass vocational issues for people with mental illness, school-based practice, and issues related to practice in rural and remote areas. In this term students also write a scholarly paper that addresses a broad aspect of the social, political, legal, or ethical environment which has a potential impact on occupational therapy practice. Often, these issues are relevant to community-based practice. In the professional roles and experiential practice (PREP) course, students are introduced to skills required for a variety of approaches to assessment, including workplace, home, and community assessments. They review non-standardized and standardized community assessments.

Term 3: Disability, Development, and Occupation

Through review of disability and rehabilitation, students gain knowledge of models of disability, including the medical model, and the independent living movement, which is grounded in community contexts. They are also introduced to a recovery-based mental health system. Skills addressed in the PREP course correspond to this, so that students are introduced to the principles of psychosocial rehabilitation and supported employment, both of which frequently involve consultation and liaison within community settings. Within the PREP class, students are also exposed to some of the initial skills important to occupational therapy in consultation and mediation roles. Other areas of community emphasis include workplace interventions, home modifications, and promoting living skills. In the problem-based tutorial component of the term, the scenarios include an occupational therapist consulting to a community addictions program to establish a life skills program, a man with a work-related repetitive strain injury, and an occupational therapist working with a woman with Pick's disease through a day hospital setting.

One student evaluation in the term that involves community linkages includes a mini-qualitative research project during which students conduct either an in-depth interview with someone experiencing a disability, or participant observation of a setting that pertains to individuals with disability, using either a phenomenological or ethnographic tradition. Regardless of the tradition, students are exposed to issues related to living with disability in the context of community.

Term 4: Youth and the Development of Self

With an emphasis on childhood and adolescence, there are a number of topics addressed within the term which are relevant to community occupational therapy practice, including family-centered service models, school-based service delivery, and transitions to adulthood. A session with ethics as a focus addresses concepts of community and students are challenged to consider the differences between groups and communities. Further opportunities for knowledge development are offered through the problem-based tutorial scenarios, which include a focus on home-based occupational therapy for an infant, school-based service for a child with challenging behaviors, and adolescent suicide. Skills addressed in the PREP course include consultation, suicide assessment, and planning and running groups. One assignment involves students conducting a developmental assessment with a typically developing child. In the evidence-based practice seminar course, students are linked up with community clinicians to conduct a search and review of evidence on a specific topic. This assignment is also discussed in the chapter on evidence-based practice.

Term 5: Adulthood and Disability

By term 5, students are well-placed to address more complex issues related to community practice and community health. The large group seminar course focuses on the roles of occupational therapists as facilitators of collaborative community development. This course builds upon the idea of practice *with* communities rather than solely *in* communities. Similarly, more complex community scenarios are presented through the problem-based tutorial scenarios including a newspaper editorial written by a woman with a disability facing issues related to returning home; a community-based social support team working with an older homeless man; an occupational therapist working as part of an assertive community treatment team; an aboriginal woman with HIV; and an occupational therapist in a case management role with a geriatric psychiatry team. In this course, students are also required to write a scholarly paper that involves exploring an occupational challenge facing a specific community and the role of occupational therapy in working with the community.

The PREP course places a similar emphasis on skills for community practice. Students review education and learning theory, and apply this through an assignment that involves consultation to develop educational materials in partnership with a community or organization. Other students are involved in using consultation skills to conduct either a community-based environmental assessment or a seating assessment and intervention plan.

Term 6: Complexities of Contemporary Practice

In the final term of study, students conduct a number of assignments that are related to making the transition into practice as occupational therapists. Many of the areas addressed include further knowledge and skill development for community practice. One assignment involves the development of a program proposal or business plan, which includes a needs assessment and an implementation and evaluation plan. This assignment is similar to the one described by Miller and Nelson (2004), although it does not have the formal community linkages as a required component. In the problem-based tutorial course in term 6, students develop their own problem scenarios based on their learning needs. The scenarios developed within each group must address a variety of practice environments, professional roles, and developmental stages. In this term the students also complete their evidence-based research projects, many of which are located in community organizations.

Curriculum Overview

Issues of community practice and community health are integrated across the occupational therapy curriculum, enabling faculty to build on the content from one term to the next. As noted in the first year of the program, students are introduced to the premises underlying community health at its broadest, while many examples provide them with opportunities to gain knowledge and skill to provide service in a variety of communities. As the students progress to the second year of the program, scenarios to which they are exposed become more complex, enabling and challenging students to consider roles that they may take as occupational therapists working with communities. Throughout the program, students are also provided with practicum experiences. Few students complete the program without having had at least one practicum in a community setting and with the increasing number of role-emerging practica, many will have the opportunity to explore occupational therapy with communities. The intent of the curricula is to provide students with opportunities to develop the knowledge, skills, and professional behaviors so that they are able to take on a variety of roles in and with communities.

Challenges Related to Community and Community Health in the Occupational Therapy Curriculum

There are challenges associated with integrating community practice and community health across the curriculum. In many circumstances, students are exposed to issues related to community practice and community health; however, if the issues are in the context of a clinical scenario, students may not pick up on the richness and complexities associated with community. This is common in the problem-based tutorial scenarios, in which for example issues of cultural diversity are often raised. However, without the client actually present, it can be very difficult for students to gain appreciation for the complexity of community practice with a client from a different cultural background. It can also be challenging to ensure that students are considering the application of skills in a community context. Within the classroom setting, it is possible to discuss the challenges and benefits of home, workplace, and community assessments, but the strategies and skills needed to successfully assess those settings can be difficult to convey. Finally, many students seem to experience challenges in appreciating the distinctions between working with individuals and communities. It is difficult to convey to students the need to think of applying skills of facilitation to community meetings, or the need to negotiate action plans with a diverse community. While some students may oversimplify the translation of skills from individuals to groups, others have a difficult time understanding the contributions that occupational therapists can make at the level of working with the community.

To address these challenges, the faculty have identified a need to communicate frequently about the content details of some sessions and problem-based tutorial scenarios, so that we can build on the work from previous units even if completely different faculty are involved from one unit to the next. Although this can be time-consuming, it is essential to ensure that students are provided with exposure to the knowledge and skills required of competent community occupational therapists.

Conclusion

This chapter has provided an overview of the distinct ways in which the Physiotherapy and Occupational Therapy Programs at McMaster University have incorporated community health and community practice into their curricula. While the content is integrated across the two years of the Occupational Therapy Program, the Physiotherapy Program has concentrated this material into one unit. In large part, the differences in the ways in which the material is organized in the curricula reflect the history and current practices of the professions. Although the organization of the curricula is different, similarities are also apparent. Both programs work to incorporate roles of consultation, education, and mediation, as well as direct service delivery in a variety of community contexts. Each works to ensure that students are provided with adequate background in theories and models of community health, public health, and global health issues. Although there are challenges in ensuring that faculty, tutors, and students are provided with adequate support to enable the development of knowledge and skills, each program has developed strategies to prepare students to graduate, prepared for evolving roles for rehabilitation professionals in community health.

References

Accreditation Council for Canadian Academic Programs, Canadian Alliance of Physiotherapy Regulators, Canada Physiotherapy Association, and Canadian University Physical Therapy Academic Council (2004) Essential competency profile. National Physiotherapy Advisory Group, Ottawa

Adams CB, Wilkins R (1992) Development of health expectancy indicators: meeting of the international network on health expectancy (REVES). Health Rep 4:67–72

Ajzen I, Fishbein M (1980) Understanding attitudes and predicting social behaviour. Prentice Hall, Englewood Cliffs, NJ

American Diabetes Association National Institute of Diabetes, and Digestive and Kidney Diseases (2003) The prevention or delay of type 2 diabetes. Diabetes Care 26:S62–S69

American Physical Therapy Association (1997a) Guide to physical therapy practice. Phys Ther 77:1163–1650

American Physical Therapy Association (1997b) A normative model of physical therapist. Professional education version 9.7. American Physical Therapy Association, Alexandria, VA

Anderson CA, Green WL (1986) Community health. Times Mirror/Mosby College Publishing, St Louis, MO

Baltes PB, Baltes MM (1990) Psychological perspectives on successful aging: the model of selective optimization with compensation. In: Baltes PB, Baltes MM (eds) Successful aging: perspectives from the behavioural sciences. Cambridge University Press, New York, NY, pp 1–34

Baltes PB, Carstensen LL (1996) The process of successful ageing. Ageing Soc 16:397–422

Bandura A (1977a) Self efficacy: the exercise of control. Freeman, New York, NY

Bandura A (1977b) Self-efficacy: toward a unifying theory of behaviour change. Psychol Rev 84:191–215

Bandura A (1986) A social cognitive theory. Prentice Hall, Engelwood Cliffs, NJ

Banks S, Head B (2004) Partnering occupational therapy and community development. Can J Occup Ther 71:5–11

Brown M, Binder EF, Korht WM (2000) Physical and performance measures for the identification of mild to moderate frailty. J Gerontol A Biol Sci Med Sci 55A:M350–M355

Bulmer M (1987) The social basis of community care. Allen and Unwin, London

Canadian Association of Occupational Therapists (1999) CAOT membership statistics 1999–2000. http://www.caot.ca/pdfs/1999-2000Stats.pdf. Retrieved 28 September 2004

Canadian Association of Occupational Therapists (2000a) Position statement on home care. Can J Occup Ther 67:351–352

Canadian Association of Occupational Therapists (2000b) Position statement on primary health care. Can J Occup Ther 67:356–358

Canadian Association of Occupational Therapists (2003a) Position statement: occupational therapy and active living for older adults. Can J Occup Ther 70:183–184

Canadian Association of Occupational Therapists (2003b) Position statement: universal design and occupational therapy. Can J Occup Ther 70:187–188

Canadian Association of Occupational Therapists (2004a) Position statement: healthy occupations for children and youth. Can J Occup Ther 71:182–183

Canadian Association of Occupational Therapists (2004b) Position statement: workplace health and occupational therapy. Can J Occup Ther 71:186–187

Canadian Working Group on HIV and Rehabilitation (2000) Report summary: policy issues on rehabilitation in the context of HIV disease: a background and position paper. Wellesley Central Hospital, Toronto

Chiu AY, Au-Yeung SS, Lo SK (2003) A comparison of four functional tests in discriminating fallers from non-fallers in older people. Disabil Rehabil 25:45–50

Christiansen CH, Townsend EA (2004) The occupational nature of communities. In: Christiansen CH, Townsend EA (eds) Introduction to occupation: the art and science of living. Prentice Hall, Upper Saddle River, NJ, pp 141–172

Colvez A, Blanchett M (1983) Potential gains in life expectancy free of disability: a tool for health planning. Int J Epidemiol 12:224–229

Commission on Accreditation in Physical Therapy Education (1998) Evaluative criteria for accreditation of education programs for the preparation of physical therapists. American Physical Therapy Association, Alexandria, VA

8

Covinsky KE, Eng C, Lui LY, Sands LP, Yaffe K (2003) The last two years of life: functional trajectories of frail older people. J Am Geriatr Soc 51:492–498

Daniel M, Gamble D (1995) Diabetes and Canada's aboriginal peoples: the need for primary prevention. Int J Nurs Stud 32:243–259

Drevdahl D (1995) Coming to voice: the power of emancipatory community interventions. Adv Nurs Sci 18:13–24

Dudgeon BJ, Greenberg SL (1998) Preparing students for consultation roles and systems. Am J Occup Ther 52:801–809

Emmons KM, Rollnick S (2001) Motivational interviewing in health care settings. Am J Prev Med 20:68–74

Finlayson M, Edwards J (1997) Evolving health environments and occupational therapy: definitions, descriptions and opportunities. Br J Occup Ther 60:70–75

Fletcher RH, Fletcher SW, Wagner EH (1982) Clinical epidemiology: the essentials. Williams and Wilkins, Baltimore, MD

Frame PS (1996) Developing a health maintenance schedule. In: Woolf SH, Jonas S (eds) Health promotion and disease prevention in clinical practice. Williams and Wilkins, Baltimore, MD, pp 467–482

Fried LP, Bandeen-Roche K, Williamson JD, Prasada-Rao P, Chee E, Rubin GS (1996) Functional decline in older adults: expanding the methods of ascertainment. J Gerontol A Biol Sci Med Sci 51A:M206–M214

Fried LP, Herdman SJ, Khun KE, et al (2001a) Preclinical disability: hypotheses about the bottom of the iceberg. J Aging Health 47:747–760

Fried LP, Tangen CM, Walston J, et al (2001b) Frailty in older adults: evidence for a phenotype. J Gerontol A Biol Sci Med Sci 56A:M146–M156

Fries J (1987) An introduction to the compression of morbidity. Gerontol Perspect 8:5–19

Gahimer JE, Morris DM (1999) Community health education. J Phys Ther Educ 13:38–48

Gill TM, Hardy SE, Williams S (2002) Underestimation of disability in community-living older persons. J Am Geriatr Soc 50:1492–1497

Golden NH (2002) A review of the female athlete triad (amenorrhea, osteoporosis and disordered eating). Int J Adolesc Med Health 14:9–17

Hamerman D (1999) Toward an understanding of frailty. Ann Intern Med 130:945–950

Hanley AJG, Harris S, Barnie A, Gittlesohn J, Wolever TM, Logan A, et al (1996) The Sandy Lake health and diabetes project: design, methods and lessons learned. Chronic Dis Can 16:149–156

Harris S, Gittelsohn J, Hanley AJG, Barnie A, Wolever TM, Gad J, et al (1997) The prevalence of NIDDM and associated risk factors in Native Canadians. Diabetes Care 20:185–187

Harris S, Hugi M, Olivotto I, Niesen-Vertommen S, Dingee C, Eddy F, et al (2001) Upper extremity rehabilitation in women with breast cancer after axillary dissection: clinical practice guidelines. Crit Rev Phys Rehabil Med 13:91–103

Health Canada (2002) Population health approach. http://hc-sc.gc.ca/hppb/phdd. Retrieved 26 Sept 2004

Herzog TA, Abrams DB, Emmons KM, Linnan L, Shadel WG (1999) Do processes of change predict smoking stage movement? A prospective analysis of the transtheoretical model. Health Psychol 4:369–375

Hutchings T, Wizowski L (2004) Developing and using patient education materials. In: 2nd year physiotherapy students (eds) Hamilton Health Sciences, Hamilton, ON

Institute of Medicine (1988) The future of public health. National Academy of Medicine, Washington, DC

Jensen GM, Lorish CD (1994) Promoting patient cooperation with exercise programs. Arthritis Care Res 7:181–189

Lai JC, Woo J, Hui E, Chan WM (2004) Telerehabilitation: a new model for community-based stroke rehabilitation. J Telemed Telecare 10:199–205

LaLonde M (1974) New perspectives on the health of Canadians. Ministry of National Health and Welfare, Ottawa, ON

Landry MD, Nixon S, Zakus D (2002) The role of the physical therapist in global health: a SWOT analysis. Department of Physical Therapy and Centre for International Health, Faculty of Medicine, University of Toronto

Last JM (1998) Social and behavioural determinants of health. In: Last JM (ed) Public health and human ecology, 2nd edn. Appleton and Lange, Stamford, CT, pp 231–268

Lee K (2004) Globalisation: what is it and how does it affect health? Med J Aust 180:156–158

Letts L, Fraser B, Finlayson M, Walls J (1993) For the health of it! Occupational therapy within a health promotion framework. CAOT Publications ACE, Toronto, ON

Lorig K, Associates (2001) Patient education: a practical approach, 3rd edn. Sage, London, p 185

Lott SA, Binkley J (2004) The role of physiotherapy related to breast cancer. Turning Point Women's Healthcare, Dahlonega, GA

Lunney JR, Lynn J, Foley DJ, Lipson S, Guralnik JM (2003) Patterns of decline at the end of life. JAMA 289:2387–2392

Manton KG (1988) A longitudinal study of functional change and mortality in the United States. J Gerontol 43:S153–S161

Martin PC, Fell DW (1999) Beyond treatment: patient education for health promotion and disease prevention. J Phys Ther Educ 13:49–56

McComas J, Carswell A (1994) A model for action in health promotion: a community experience. Can J Rehabil 7:257–265

Megens A, Harris S (1998) Physical therapist management of lymphedema following treatment for breast cancer: a critical review of its effectiveness. Phys Ther 78:1302–1311

Miller BK, Nelson D (2004) Constructing a program development proposal for community-based practice: a valuable learning experience for occupational therapy students. Occup Ther Health Care 18:137–150

Miller WR, Rollnick S (2002) Motivational interviewing: preparing people for change. Guildford Press, New York, NY

Minkler M (1999) Personal responsibility for health? A review of the arguments and the evidence at century's end. Health Educ Behav 26:121–140

Moreland J, Richardson J, Chan D, O'Neill J, Bellissimo A, Grum R, et al (2003) Evidence-based guidelines for the secondary prevention of falls in older adults. Gerontology 49:93–116

Olshansky SJ, Ault AB (1986) The fourth stage of the epidemiology transition, the age of delayed degenerative diseases. Milbank Q 64:355–391

Omran AR (1971) The epidemiologic transition: a theory of epidemiology of population change. Millbank Q 49:509–538

Patrick WK, Cadman EC (2002) Changing emphases in public health and medical education in health care reform. Asia Pac J Public Health 14:35–39

Patrick DL, Curtis JR, Engleburg RA, Nilesen E, McCowan E (2003) Measuring and improving the quality of dying and death. Ann Intern Med 139:410–415

Penninx BW, Leveille S, Ferrucci L, van Eijk JT, Guralnik JM (1999) Exploring the effect of depression on physical disability: longitudinal evidence from the established populations for epidemiologic studies of the elderly. Am J Public Health 39:1346–1352

Penninx BW, Deeg DJ, van Eijk JT, Beekman AT, Guralnik JM (2000) Changes in depression and functional decline in older adults: a longitudinal perspective. J Affect Disord 61:1–12

Prochaska JO, DiClemente CC (1983) Stages and processes of self-change of smoking: toward an integrative model of change. J Consult Clin Psychol 51:390–395

Prochaska JO, Redding C, Evers K (1997) The transtheoretical model and stages of change. Jossey-Bass, San Francisco, CA

Riddle DL, Stratford PW (1999) Interpreting validity indexes for diagnostic tests: an illustration of the Berg balance test. Phys Ther 79:939–948

Rogers R, Hackenberg R (1987) Epidemiologic transition theory. Soc Biol 34:234–243

Rosenstock IM, Kirscht JP (1974) The health belief model and personal health behaviour. Health Education Monogr 2:470–473

Rowe J, Khan RL (1987) Human aging: usual and successful. Science 237:143–149

Sabatini S (2001) The female athlete triad: a review. Am J Med Sci 322:193–195

Scaffa ME (2001) Community based practice: occupation in context. In: Scaffa ME (ed) Occupational therapy in community-based practice settings. Davis, Philadelphia, PA, pp 3–18

Shinitzky H, Kub J (2001) The art of motivational behaviour change: the use of motivational interviewing to promote health. Public Health Nurs 18:178–185

Statistics Canada (2002) Disability-free life expectancy at age 65 by sex, Canada, province, territories, health regions and peer groups. Health Indicators Catalogue 82 221-XIE 5:1–6

Strecher VJ, de Vellis BM, Becker MH, Rosenstock IM (1997) The health belief model. In: Glanz K, Lewis FM, Rimmer BK (eds) Health behaviour and health education: theory, research and practice. Jossey-Bass, San Francisco, CA

Sutton S (1996) Can "stages of change" provide guidance in the treatment of addictions? A critical examination of Prochaska and DiClemente's model. In: Edwards G, Dare C (eds) Psychotherapy, psychological treatments and the addictions. Cambridge University Press, Cambridge, pp 189–205

Thibeault R, Hebert M (1997) A congruent model of health promotion in occupational therapy. Occup Ther Int 4:271–293

Tinnetti ME, Baker DI, McAvay G, Claus EB, Garret P, Gottschalk, et al (1994) A multifactorial intervention to reduce the risk of falling among elderly people living in the community. N Engl J Med 331:821–827

Van de Water HP, Perenboom RJ (1996) Policy relevance of the health expectancy indicator and inventory in European Union countries. Health Policy 36:117–129

Von Korff M, Ormel J, Katon W, Lin EH (1992) Disability and depression among high utilizers of health care: a longitudinal analysis. Arch Gen Psychiatry 49:91–100

West VR (1998) The female athlete triad: the triad of disordered eating, amenorrhoea and osteoporosis. Sports Med 26:63–71

Wilson JF (2003) The crucial link between literacy and health. Ann Intern Med 139:875–878

Wizowski L, Harper T, Hutchings T (2002) Writing health information for patients and families: a guide to creating patient education materials that are easy to read, understand and use. Hamilton Health Sciences, Hamilton, Ontario

World Health Organization (1986) Ottawa charter for health promotion. Paper presented at the International Conference on Health Promotion, Ottawa, 17–21 Nov 1986

World Health Organization (2001) International classification of functioning, disability and health. Author, Geneva

Chapter 9

Developing Communication Skills

9

Sue Baptiste, Patricia Solomon

Contents

All professional preparation programs require that their graduates develope strong skills in communicating with clients, colleagues, employers, and others of significance in the practice environment. However, since the mid 1990s, there have been several major trends developing that place an additional emphasis upon the need for in-depth education in the area of communication skills. Many of these trends have been mentioned already in this book, but bear repetition in the context of teaching and engendering exemplary communication skills in our graduates.

Radical changes in organizational models have created working environments within which there is a specific demand for individual clinicians to become assertive and to practice from a sense of professional autonomy and purpose. Within such environments, it is imperative that practitioners feel confident and able to communicate clearly and with firm intention in order for their practice philosophy and mission to become realized within the work place.

There are increased expectations for supervision of support personnel, either those with specific training in rehabilitation or others of a more generic nature. This requires abilities to communicate clearly in written and verbal ways and to also exhibit skills in negotiation, delegation, and conflict resolution.

Opportunities for becoming involved in newly emerging roles are becoming commonplace, thereby offering new graduates and seasoned therapists alike the chance to strike out into new territory. Although this is an exciting reality, there are associated expectations for clarity in professional role and focus, thus putting skills in imparting opinion, feedback, and information to the test.

Overall, there is an overarching need to communicate with a broad range of people: clients, families, other professionals, managers, government representatives, politicians, researchers, policy makers and planners, and so forth. There is less time to create a supportive treatment environment and, therefore, the need to streamline rapport-building skills is of paramount importance within professional preparation curricula. While teaching communication skills has always had its place within health professional education programs, there has been a recent need to review and revamp these programs with a view to insuring that there is congruence between communication style and client-centered principles. With the emergence of a client-centered approach to delivering health care services, building relationships with clients has become more a matter of creating partnerships than simply imparting expertise and information. There is also a growing need to practice in a manner that is respectful and sensitive to cultural differences, given the multicultural nature of societies around the world.

Elements of Communication Skills

Communication skills are important to every field in the health sciences, and since the late 1990s have been given specific attention. A 1999 international consensus statement on communications teaching and assessment in medical education provided several clear and helpful recommendations that apply readily across the full sphere of health sciences education (Makoul and Schofield 2001). Curriculum content centered upon the teaching and evaluation of communication skills should be based on a broad view of this area incorporating communication skills development throughout the academic and clinical experiential components of the curriculum in a complementary and consistent fashion. Students should be helped to develop sound client-centered communication skills, in congruence with enhancing self-awareness thus enriching personal and professional growth. There should be a planned and coherent framework with the learners' ability to achieve communication tasks assessed directly by observation and experiential opportunities. Communication skills teaching and assessment programs should be evaluated as with any other element of a curricular model, and faculty development should be considered an essential component of the whole (Makoul and Schofield 2001).

Much of the most recent work exploring the critical importance of communication and self-awareness skills for health professionals resides within the medical educational network and emerging literature. Several accrediting bodies, such as the Association of American Medical Colleges (AAMC), the General Medical Council (GMC), and the Accreditation Council for Graduate Medical Education (ACGME), have expressed the importance of communication skills to good healthcare practice, linking it closely to professional behaviors (Makoul 2003a; Whitcomb 2000). Provider–patient/client communication has been given the most attention in the area of educating for communication skills, primarily because it is believed that poor communication can negatively affect patient compliance and outcomes, and an effective approach to communicating with patients and families can do the opposite (Barrier et al. 2003; Chant et al. 2002b; Lubbers and Roy 1990; Maguire and Pitceathly 2002; Yedidia et al. 2003). As Gadacz (2003) illustrates, poor communication skills can also have a deleterious effect on other relationships the provider might have, such as with colleagues or other medical personnel. Scientific and technological advances in medicine have placed an increased burden on health care students (providers in training) to assimilate vast amounts of knowledge; in the process, interpersonal interactions that have previously been learned at the bedside or within the direct practice setting have been de-emphasized. All too often practitioners are faced with the problem of feeling that they do not have enough time to spend listening to clients and showing compassion for their circumstances. Expectations of funders and supervisors that a prescribed number of patients/clients will be seen within a working day seems to challenge and defeat the professional mission. Communication skills must therefore be taught explicitly, in a manner that fits well into current and evolving curricula, and must incorporate both skills of communicating and being self-aware (Morgan and Winter 1996).

What is taught or imparted in the name of communication skills is currently under great scrutiny. Much of the impetus for this attention is due to the recognition that working relationships within health care teams and agencies cannot be assumed to be collaborative. Also, changing conceptual models of health care delivery are pointing more and more to the centrality of relationships in the search for the most responsive delivery options and optimal outcomes (Foss 1996). A major focus of research on communication skills teaching has been on the medical interview, including identifying the key elements of an effective interview. The American Academy on Physician and Patient (AAPP) adopted a framework for this interview, within which there are three functions: information gathering, relationship building, and patient education (Barrier et al. 2003). Maguire and Pitceathly (2002) have added the element of "being supportive" to this list. When feelings, thoughts, and experiences are reduced to "skills" and the complex, multilayered interaction between people are reduced to "behaviors", a much greater emphasis is placed upon the seen than the unseen (Zoppi and Epstein 2002). Too much emphasis on observable behaviors can lead students to believe that it is sufficient to go through the motions of patient-centered interviewing (mechanistic communication) without being a truly attentive and responsive listener (relational communication) (Chant et al. 2002b; Zoppi and Epstein 2002).

Certainly, the essence of this framework can readily be transposed to the educational and training needs of other disciplines, including occupational therapy and physiotherapy. It is now being recognized that non-verbal cues can be just as important to patient–provider communication as the words spoken. Efforts should thus be made to teach students about the importance of paralanguage, physical appearance, facial expression, visual behavior, touch, space, time, and environmental cues (Makoul 2003b).

Teaching and Evaluating Communication Skills

In the Occupational Therapy and Physiotherapy Programs at McMaster University, our approach to imparting the essential elements of communication skills and self-awareness has been well grounded in the foundational educational philosophy of problem-based learning.

It has become evident that in many cases, evaluation tends to drive learning. Evaluating communication skills within the curriculum makes explicit the importance and value of this aspect of health care practice. The *Objective Structured Clinical Examination* (OSCE) has been reviewed as an effective way of measuring communication skills (Yedidia et al. 2003). Other ways of evaluating student learning related to communication skills are many and varied. The *use of video or audiotapes* to provide evidence of accomplishment provides a self-assessment measure and an opportunity for an external observer to provide expert input and a formative or summative rating. Similarly the use of *patient simulations* is very valuable, including asking the "patient" to provide structured feedback to the learner face-to-face and in writing. Students can be expected to complete a self-rating and a *self-assessment* through reflection in writing or in person with a faculty advisor or mentor. Within the direct practice environment, during fieldwork or experiential opportunities, feedback from patients/clients and families can be sought to complement the feedback given by the clinical preceptor or supervisor. While communications skills are teachable, and can be learned in a theoretical manner, teaching is most effective when there is an *integrated application of these skills during clinical experiences* across several different environments and patient populations (Aspegren 1999; Yedidia et al. 2003). An emphasis on lifelong learning also helps to narrow the theory–practice gap (Chant et al. 2002a) and is a natural part of a problem-based learning environment. *Portfolios* and workbooks also encourage reflection (Chant et al. 2002b).

Faculty development is vital in the teaching of communication skills, as many faculty members are not trained to teach in this area. As with any identifiable curriculum component, formal faculty development will ensure effective guidance and feedback to students on their performance (Yedidia et al. 2003). It also helps faculty improve their own communication skills, which is vital considering the importance of *role modeling* in the acquisition of practice skills for students (Laidlaw et al. 2002; Maguire and Pitceathly 2002).

Illustrations from McMaster University

Video, Audiotapes, and Standardized Patients in Simulated Interviews and Practice Interactions

Students require some kind of sounding board through which they may receive feedback on how they appear to others as they attempt to establish a professional persona that is congruent with who they are as a person. This can be achieved through engaging in simulated interviews, being observed in the process and also by recording the experience in some way. Standardized patients are individuals who have been trained to reflect a specific patient/client situation and to respond in character throughout an interview with a health sciences learner. These people are trained to stay in role during the course of the formal interview period and then to provide feedback to the student using a structured protocol. Both the occupational therapy and physiotherapy programs use standardized patients widely throughout the curriculum starting in the first study unit. Taping or recording is used less frequently, and often is employed more when remediation is required for a particular student. Remediation is when a student has not completed a course or assignment successfully and has been granted the opportunity to re-do this element of the program. In these circumstances, being able to view one's own behaviors can be an invaluable way in which to understand the areas of weakness requiring attention.

For example, in term 1 of the occupational therapy program, two focused sessions are provided to students that address interviewing skills from the perspective of a definite model and its application in practice. In the first session, the students participate in an interviewing exercise in groups of three, during which they experiment with their understanding of interviewing. The session objective is to demonstrate the ability to communicate effectively with clients and colleagues, and includes being able to identify the therapist, client, and environmental factors that enhance or impede therapeutic communication and the demonstration of interviewing, giving constructive feedback and identifying gaps in information. After the students have attempted their interview experience, information is shared concerning the important elements of communicating in an interview context, including:

- Therapeutic communication
- Dimensions of communication
- Verbal and non-verbal communications
- Enablers and barriers in communications and strategies to ameliorate these concerns
- Empathy and sympathy
- Active listening

The second session provides an opportunity to review the material presented previously and to introduce the students to interviewing that is more focused on occupational therapy practice. Information is provided concerning instruments that will help to name, validate, and prioritize occupational performance issues, such as the Canadian Occupational Performance Measure (Law et al. 1991, 1994). Prior to the end of the session, all students engage in pairs in a short practice exercise using a problem scenario as the context of the interview. They each assume the role of interviewer or client and are encouraged to change roles if time permits.

While interviewing skills alone do not constitute the communication skills curriculum, there is a clear focus upon the acquisition of such basic interactional skills within the first study term in the occupational therapy program. Students are required to complete two interviews during the course of these first four months in the program. In addition, their clinical practicum experience is focused upon observing professional and practice behaviors within a real world setting, and also requires them to interview patients and to assess their own performance, recording their thoughts and insights in a journal format.

In physiotherapy, students interview standardized patients early in the first unit to highlight and reinforce the importance of communication skills. We have found that in the early stages of their education, physiotherapy students often approach the interview from a purely diagnostic perspective and ask many questions related to the mechanism of injury and characteristics of pain. By conducting interviews with standardized patients who have come to them with a diagnosis (e.g., post-fractured hip) and who are experiencing difficulties related to psychosocial circumstances (e.g., depressed, worried about caring for grandchildren) they quickly learn to appreciate the importance of a client-centered approach, of understanding the "problem" from the patient's perspective and of developing a positive relationship with the patient. Many students find this exercise to be difficult, so we have found it is important to debrief from the sessions in large groups discussing what was challenging and/or surprising and strategies to facilitate communication. Standardized patients have many other advantages, including providing feedback to students on their communication style and allowing students to practice their skills in a safe environment.

Self-assessment and Self-awareness

As mentioned earlier when reflecting on the current medical education literature, a commitment to gaining self-awareness and engaging in ongoing self-assessment are two essential elements of truly communicating with patients, clients, families, and colleagues. Students within our programs at McMaster University are encouraged, facilitated, and expected to engage at an early stage in understanding themselves well, and coming to terms with their own values, biases, and strengths. Within the occupational therapy program, this complex task is accomplished through many various means, but with the expectation that each student will complete a Personal Portfolio. There is a structure given to the students for the development of the portfolio, and this includes listings of what to include as well as key questions along the continuum of the program. The portfolio is expected to include reflections upon evaluations completed, assessments undergone, and so on.

In the first term of the occupational therapy program, students are asked to complete a short, personal reflective paper on the meaning of "occupation" to them. They choose two situations in which they are engaged: firstly, an occupation that was meaningful to them and secondly, another situation where the occupation was not meaningful at all. Through a process of self-reflection, each student compares and contrasts the two chosen occupations and distills from that process the key elements of meaning for themselves. They then relate it to the meaning for future clients and how this learning has helped them to appreciate the unique nature of meaning for everyone. Later on, toward the end of the curriculum, they are asked to re-read this paper, and to think about how they view the same question from the position of being close to graduation and entry to practice.

During the first term of both programs, the students work together on "Exploring Perspectives on Disability". A group of community volunteers agree to spend time with pairs of students (one from each of the disciplines) for the students to observe the impact of disability on their lives and the strategies they use to deal with their disabilities. The volunteers are from all ages and have a wide range of abilities and disabilities. The students attend a large group session to explore the concept of disability at which time they receive the name of their volunteer. Each student pair is responsible for contacting their volunteer to arrange a time of at least two hours when they will meet together. Activities could include interviewing the volunteer or participating in activities within the individual's home or in the broader community that demonstrate the experience of living with a disability.

Also in the first term of the occupational therapy program, the students participate in an inquiry session within which they explore notions of culture, ethics, and spirituality. A model has been developed that incorporates these three complex constructs, linking personal, professional, and societal elements of professional development. Spirituality is linked to the personal, ethics to the professional, and culture to society. Through this model, students explore their own sense of self and their understanding of their chosen discipline within society by addressing some fundamental questions of who they are, where they came from, what they believe in, what they value, and how they view right and wrong. This process is accomplished through the use of dialogue in pairs, small groups, and the large group. As with many, if not all, interactional processes in problem-based learning environments, the use of narrative in communicating with each other is seen as essential and central. This process helps in highlighting the need for understanding others in a way that is sensitive to difference and celebratory of diversity. These skills addressed at an early stage of the development of a professional identity serve to lay a strong foundation for a future practice style that values listening and working collaboratively with clients and families.

Peer Tutoring to Promote Communication Skills

A tutor in a small group, problem-based environment requires communication and group facilitation and evaluation skills that are useful in a variety of professional roles. In the physiotherapy program, faculty developed a unique peer tutoring model to assist students in acquiring these skills. Previous literature suggests that students' learning is not compromised when participating in peer tutoring educational events (Andersen et al. 1996; DeGrave et al. 1990; Johansen et al. 1992; Moust and Schmidt 1993; Sorbal 1994). It was our hope that the peer tutoring experience would help students to acquire communication skills that would be useful in their future careers.

During the final unit of study, each student is responsible for facilitating a tutorial group as they work through one problem scenario (Solomon and Crowe 1999, 2001). This typically requires the student to facilitate two or three sessions. While students are familiar with problem-based learning and have experienced a variety of different tutorial groups and tutor styles throughout their education at McMaster University, they have not had the opportunity to assume the role of tutor. Faculty assuming a new tutoring role will generally undergo a two-day period of training and apprenticeship with an experienced tutor. This is not feasible for 50 to 60 students. However, students are provided with introductory training via a two-hour workshop. The workshop focuses on the fundamentals of basic facilitation skills, including an awareness of how different types of questions elicit different information, strategies for monitoring group process, and how the timing of interventions can influence both group dynamics and problem-solving. We are also cognizant of the literature that suggests the ideal tutor is one who is both content expert and has expert tutor skills (e.g., Dolmans et al. 2001). While students are not to become instant content experts, we want to ensure that they have an opportunity to familiarize themselves with the content and objectives of the problem prior to their tutoring experience. As a result each peer tutor is required to attend a tutors' meeting designed to provide background knowledge on the problem. The faculty member who developed the problem meets with peer tutors to review the specific content to be emphasized, answer any questions, and provide key resources to the peer tutors. There is also a faculty tutor assigned to each group whose role is to be a resource to the student tutor and the group, to facilitate group function and maximize student learning, to be supportive of student autonomy, and to promote individual and group evaluation.

Ongoing evaluation of this model from the student peer tutors' and faculty tutors' perspectives has resulted in changes over time. Initially faculty members struggled with their role, unsure of how directive to be in the presence of the peer tutor. Some faculty who were accustomed to the traditional tutor role felt a need to be active during the sessions. It is important that faculty have a clear understanding of their role since if they were too directive during the process, the peer tutor's performance may be undermined. Students worry that they may not master the content of the tutorial when they assume the peer tutor role. Faculty tutors need to work with the student groups so that the students value the learning inherent in assuming the tutor role and feel confident that they are mastering the relevant content. This is often difficult in a final unit of study where students are focused upon the upcoming professional licensing examinations.

Overall, the students evaluate these experiences very positively. Students enjoy the role; many find this experience motivates them to return to the program to tutor following graduation. As a part of the process of evaluation, each student is asked to write a reflective journal outlining their experiences as a peer tutor, including their personal objectives, their strengths and weaknesses, and any other perceptions. While there are many insights into the learning that occurred it is evident that much of the learning relates to communication skills. Many reflect on specific situations in which their tutoring skills would be helpful:

>> These skills would be helpful when empowering clients by asking questions that let them come up with ideas and solutions to problems rather than be dictating answers. (Solomon and Crowe 1999 p. 201)

When in family conferences, I will be able to encourage family problem-solving and critical thinking. (Solomon and Crowe 1999 p. 201)

Students are able to see the relevance of the skills in future clinical practice. As one student wrote:

>> The active listening and questioning skills that are required of a tutor will also help me in team and committee meetings in the future. I feel that I will be able to listen to the contributions of others, question others to promote clarifying and make personal contributions, while being open-minded and non-threatening. (Solomon and Crowe 2001 p. 184)

Another stated:

> » Although I will not be employed as a "teacher", I will always be teaching in this field, and I can apply these skills and abilities and use them as an asset in almost any setting, personal and professional. (Solomon and Crowe 1999 p. 201)

Peer tutoring offers an innovative way for students to work on specific communication skills related to group facilitation and evaluation.

Problem-based learning is the ideal vehicle for incorporating all elements of communication skills. The experience of being in a small tutorial group provides a natural learning environment for essential skills of relationship building and team functioning. Each tutorial session is evaluated at the end of the time period, by using indicators for determining the quality of group process and the facilitation of learning that has taken place on that particular day. Each group member is expected to provide honest and thoughtful input to this conversation, with the goal of ironing out the difficulties that may have arisen, and also to recognize the positive attributes of the manner in which group members are relating and working together. This has a clear connection to what it means to work in health care teams for the purpose of providing quality health care services to clients and families. These experiences stand our students in very good stead when entering a new team situation and creating their own personal professional identity and niche. Similarly, when working within problem-based learning in small groups there is an inherent expectation for engaging in a reciprocal process of feedback. Giving and receiving constructive feedback are essential skills for anyone who will be working within a team context. Being in close proximity to peers and tutor in the process of gaining critical thinking and clinical reasoning abilities is an ideal way in which such communication skills can be learned and internalized.

The Written Word

As we have stated earlier, communication skills are not simply a matter of knowing how to engage in and complete a good client interview. Communication skills also include developing an understanding of self and a commitment to continued self-awareness and personal reflection. Similarly, the need for excellence in written communication cannot be underestimated. From clear interview notes to succinct report writing, skills in imparting information in written formats are central to successful and ethical professional practice.

From the onset of both the occupational therapy and physiotherapy programs, students are engaged in writing. They are expected to gain a high level of skill in writing academically as well as for the clinical arena. Expectations of learners include the preparation of academic and professional manuscripts that could be deemed suitable for publication at a professional level, in either newsletters or established journals. In preparation for clinical placements, there are sessions provided within the clinical skills laboratory setting for becoming familiar with the demands of chart writing. The art of summarizing clinical findings is also an expectation with the student occupational therapists completing several assessment projects related to client reports, program evaluations, and work-site/environmental assessments.

Students in both programs complete a Program Proposal or Business Plan in the last study term. This project was designed to provide the students with an opportunity to become familiar with the intricacies of writing proposals, a skill that is much in demand in many practice settings. They are provided with a framework that includes: an introduction; a needs assessment; a description of the new program, role, or practice; the resources required; an implementation plan; a program evaluation; and a conclusion and executive summary. Completed essay papers are evaluated by faculty members from the School of Rehabilitation Science who are from any discipline. Many students use these proposals as a basis for developing programs and businesses once they practice. As outlined in Chapter 8, students also develop skills related to designing patient education materials.

The Presented Word

Throughout both curricula, our students are encouraged and supported in the process of gaining strong presentation skills. From the outset of the first terms of study, students are expected to employ creative presentation models to inform peers and faculty during large group inquiry sessions, clinical skills laboratories, and in the more intimate context of their small group tutorials. In term 1 of the occupational therapy program, the students work in their tutorial groups, but within the large group inquiry seminar, to present foundational models of occupation to their peers. This is part of the learning evaluation for that course, but also an early opportunity to practice existing skills of presentation and gain new ones. This focus continues across the six study terms and culminates in all students from both programs participating in symposia in the final term at which they present the results of their evidence-based/research projects to a mixed audience of their peers, faculty, community practitioners, and significant other attendees including family and faculty from across the university who have been involved in the projects. In participating in these kinds of experiences, the students gain skill in current information technology as well as abilities of engaging an audience and delivering their message.

Conclusion

In this chapter, we have provided an overview of the manner in which we embrace and integrate the development of communication skills into our curricula in occupational therapy and physiotherapy. There is no doubt that communication skills in and of themselves are critical to the preparation of competent entry-level practitioners. Such skills take many forms – from learning how to relate to clients, families, communities, peers, and faculty to gaining more concrete skills of writing succinctly and presenting clearly at the podium. Undoubtedly, existing within a problem-based learning culture that values relationships is a bonus for the development and appreciation of communication skills in general. We recognize the particular opportunities offered by the small group and large group format of the curricula and value them.

References

Andersen R, Robins L, Fitzgerald J, Zweifler A (1996) Fourth-year medical students as small group leaders of first-year students. Acad Med 71:793–794

Aspegren K (1999) BEME guide no. 2: teaching and learning communication skills in medicine: a review with quality grading of articles. Med Teach 21:563–570

Barrier PA, Li JC, Jensen NM (2003) Two words to improve physician-patient communication: what else? Mayo Clin Proc 78:211–214

Chant S, Jenkinson T, Randle J, Russell G (2002a) Communication skills: some problems in nursing education and practice. J Clin Nurs 11:12–21

Chant S, Jenkinson T, Randle J, Russell G, Webb C (2002b) Communication skills training in healthcare: a review of the literature. Nurse Educ Today 22:189–202

DeGrave W, De Volder M, Gijselaers W, Demouiseaux V (1990) Peer teaching and problem based learning: tutor characteristics, tutor functioning, group functioning, and student achievement. In: Nooman Z, Schmidt H, Ezzat E (eds) Innovation in medical education: in the valuation of its present status. Springer, Berlin Heidelberg New York, pp 123–124

Dolmans DHJM, Wolfhagen IHAP, Scherpbier AJJA, van der Vleuten CPM (2001) Relationship of tutors' group dynamics skills to their performance ratings in problem-based learning. Acad Med 76:473–476

Foss L (1996) Advancing psychosocial health education: a review of the Pew-Fetzer report. Advances 12:43–50

Gadacz TR (2003) A changing culture in interpersonal and communication skills. Am Surg 69:453–458

Johansen M, Martensen D, Bircher J (1992) Students as tutors in problem based learning: does it work? Med Educ 26:163–165

Laidlaw T, MacLeod H, Kaufman D, Langille D, Sargeant J (2002) Implementing a communication skills programme in medical school: needs assessment and programme change. Med Educ 36:115–124

Law M, Baptiste S, Carswell-Opzoomer A, McColl M, Polatajko H, Pollock M (1991) Canadian occupational therapy performance measure manual. CAOT Publications, Toronto

Law M, Polatajko H, Pollock N, McColl MA, Carswell A, Baptiste S (1994) Pilot testing of the Canadian occupational therapy performance measure: clinical and measurement issue. Can J Occup Ther 61:191–197

Lubbers CA, Roy SJ (1990) Communication skills for continuing education in nursing. J Contin Educ Nurs 21:109–112

Maguire P, Pitceathly C (2002) Key communication skills and how to acquire them. BMJ 325:697–700

Makoul G (2003a) Communication skills education in medical school and beyond. JAMA 289:93

Makoul G (2003b) The interplay between education and research about patient-provider communication. Patient Educ Couns 50:79–84

Makoul G, Schofield T (2001) Communication teaching and assessment in medical education: an international consensus statement. Patient Educ Couns 37:191–195

Morgan ER, Winter R (1996) Teaching communication skills. an essential part of residency training. Arch Pediatr Adolesc Med 150:638–642

Moust J, Schmidt H (1993) Comparing students and faculty as tutors: how effective are they? In: Bouhuis P (ed) PBL as an educational strategy. Network Publications, Maastricht, pp 121–134

Solomon P, Crowe J (1999) Evaluation of a model of student peer tutoring. In: Conway J, Williams A (eds) Themes and variations in PB. University of Newcastle, New South Wales, Australia, pp 196–205

Solomon P, Crowe J (2001) Perceptions of student peer tutors in a problem based learning program. Med Teach 23:181–186

Sorbal D (1994) Peer tutoring and student outcomes in a problem based learning course. Med Educ 28:284–289

Whitcomb ME (2000) Communication and professionalism. Patient Educ Couns 41:137–144

Yedidia MJ, Gillespie CC, Kachur E, Schwartz MD, Ockene J, Chepaitis AE, et al (2003) Effect of communications training on medical student performance. JAMA 290:1157–1165

Zoppi K, Epstein RM (2002) Is communication a skill? Communication behaviors and being in relation. Fam Med 34:319–324

Developing Community Partnerships

10

Patricia Solomon, Sue Baptiste

Contents

One of the greatest strengths of the Occupational Therapy (OT) and Physiotherapy (PT) Programs at McMaster University is the sustained commitment of the clinical community. Accreditors, visitors, and students are consistently impressed with the approximately 120 part-time unfunded clinical faculty each of whom contribute 50–100 hours to the programs every year. However, the relationship between the community and the university is not perceived as one-sided. The goal is for the university to be a part of the professional community and work in harmony with all stakeholders to improve research, practice, and education in the rehabilitation sciences.

The model for our community partnerships reflects the values of the School of Rehabilitation Science at McMaster University. These values are founded in a culture of respect and admiration for our community partners. We believe that clinical skills and expertise are equal in importance to those skills associated with scholarly activity, and that working together promotes mutually beneficial outcomes for all involved in the educational process. Commitment to self-directed, lifelong learning is another value which influences the relationships. The university provides opportunities for clinical faculty to engage in ongoing learning opportunities and mentoring relationships to help achieve career goals. This partnership is not easy to maintain in a health care system under ever-increasing fiscal restraints and an education system with growing research and educational demands. The university must provide effective infrastructure to recruit, reward, and evaluate clinical faculty. The clinical community must value the relationship with the community and perceive that there are benefits to involvement in the university's educational and research initiatives. This chapter will describe our community–university model and the challenges and supports necessary to sustain an effective partnership.

10

Description of Clinical Faculty Positions

A description of the clinical faculty positions will place this chapter into context. At McMaster University, clinical faculty differ from "adjunct" faculty who are defined as instructors employed to teach a course or part of a course in a higher education program (Copolillo et al. 2001). The clinical faculty positions are unfunded positions in which the faculty member is employed by an institution outside of the university. These are typically, but not exclusively, clinical facilities. There are two types of appointment:

1. Part-time clinical faculty appointment
   A clinician who takes a part-time clinical faculty appointment contributes approximately 100 hours of his or her time to either the OT or PT Program each year. This is a more traditional model in which faculty members must meet specific criteria to both receive and maintain their faculty appointment. It is recognized that these faculty are primarily clinicians and they are eligible for promotion through the ranks of Clinical Lecturer, Assistant Clinical Professor, Associate Clinical Professor, and Clinical Professor. In a research-intensive university, scholarly activity is an expectation of all faculty, though in recognition of the fact that their primary responsibilities are in the clinical arena the expectations for clinical faculty are less than for tenured faculty. The performance and contributions of all clinical faculty are reviewed on a three-year basis at which time an internal committee makes decisions on reappointment and promotion to the Faculty Promotion and Tenure Committee.

2. Professional Associate Appointment

The Professional Associate appointment was developed to recognize the contributions of those who are not eligible for a "traditional" clinical faculty appointment. The clinician may not meet the minimum criteria for eligibility for a clinical faculty appointment (e.g., a masters degree and regular scholarly contributions) or be unable to contribute 100 hours to the programs on an annual basis. Each Professional Associate commits 50 hours per year to the educational programs. Professional Associates undergo a review every three years; however, the review is solely by an internal committee of the School of Rehabilitation Science.

Why Establish a Unfunded Clinical Faculty Stream?

While from the academic institution's perspective, the fact that a clinical faculty stream provides additional unfunded faculty would appear to be a powerful motivator, this is insufficient rationale for development. In the School of Rehabilitation Science the community–university partnerships are viewed as being important for the professions as a whole. The benefits are discussed below with a somewhat artificial distinction between those for the institution and those for the clinical faculty member. It must be emphasized that this is a true partnership with the goal of building mutually supporting environments. Nonetheless, it is true that the contributions of clinical faculty have allowed us to maintain a more intimate learning environment. In the School of Rehabilitation Science, the cornerstone of learning is the small group problem-based tutorial. We have found the optimal size of a tutorial group to be between 6 and 8 students. In a group of this size students are able to participate regularly and the tutor is able to provide ongoing and extensive feedback to individual students on a regular basis. In a three semester per year program with 60 students, this translates to 8–10 tutors per semester or 48–60 tutors per class over a year of study. The involvement of clinical faculty allows for the maintenance of small groups in our programs. Clinical faculty assume a wide variety of other roles including evaluator, clinical skills laboratory assistant and developer of resource materials. Table 10.1 outlines some of the typical roles and responsibilities.

Table 10.1. Examples of roles for clinical faculty

Role	Description
Problem-based tutor	Work with six or seven students twice a week for 2.5-hour session to develop and address learning issues from health care problems
Clinical skills tutor	Teach and/or evaluate student assessment and treatment skills
Guest lecturer	Provide a session on a topic in an area of clinical expertise
Committee member	Community involvement in a number of committees including admissions, curriculum, and ad hoc
Education resource	Act as a resource for a number of initiatives including development of health care problems and clinical learning experiences, assisting with student evaluation, or be available to students for consultation

The benefits to the academic institution extend far beyond enabling smaller student to faculty ratios. In a research-intensive institution it is often difficult for tenure stream faculty to maintain an active clinical caseload. Clinician involvement in all aspects of the academic program helps to maintain a current clinical perspective. A high level of clinician involvement adds credibility to the curriculum, particularly when students are concerned that academic faculty are not seeing clients and patients and hence are not "in tune" with current practices. A visible partnership between academic and clinical faculty portrays an important message to the students and helps to close the "theory–practice gap" that is often perceived by the students.

Students enjoy exposure to a wide variety of clinical and academic faculty and to varying teaching styles. In fact the involvement of the clinical community in the educational programs is consistently ranked by the students as one of the major strengths of the programs. Given the diverse nature of practice today it is unlikely that a small pool of academic faculty could provide the spectrum of skills, knowledge, and expertise that is provided through the clinical faculty stream. This is the reason many PT and OT educational programs employ clinicians as adjunct faculty. The unique aspect of the programs at McMaster University is the sheer number of clinical faculty with whom the students interact in each semester of study.

In today's ever changing and frantic health care environment one wonders why a busy clinician would be interested in assuming clinical faculty responsibilities. Tremblay et al. (2001) surveyed clinical faculty who had tutored in the OT Program at McMaster University. Those motivated to tutor enjoyed the role of educator, received pleasure through the intimacy of a small group learning environment, and felt that they had a unique perspective to offer the students. Another motivator was related to professional development; tutors found that the tutoring experience helped keep their knowledge current. About 10 percent of the tutors in the study stated that they felt tutoring was a part of their "professional obligation." Similarly, alumni of the OT and PT Programs at McMaster University often return to contribute to the educational programs. When asked informally why they want to participate, they mention the richness that the clinical faculty provided to their education and of wanting to "give something back" to the program in appreciation.

Copolillo et al. (2001) found that one of the benefits of being an adjunct OT faculty included informing and invigorating practice though the reading and reviewing of literature and following new developments in the field. Although the clinical faculty in our programs do not have the same responsibilities for curriculum development and coordination as would adjunct faculty, they also benefit from the exposure to current information. An example is related to the popular evidence-based practice (EBP) movement. The EBP movement started at McMaster University under the original name of evidence-based medicine (Evidence Based Medicine Working Group 1992) and has had a great impact on all health professional programs at the university. The expectations related to EBP for OT and PT students are high (see Chapter 5). At the beginning of the EBP movement, there were few clinical faculty who were familiar with EBP principles and their application to practice. This led to a potential problem; it could be very difficult for clinical faculty to reinforce EBP in tutorials and clinical skills laboratories if they were not confident with their knowledge. Supports have been developed to enable clinical faculty to improve their knowledge and skills with the assistance of academic faculty. For example, current and seminal articles come with supporting tutors' guides which explain in detail the learning objectives, critical content, and key facilitation points. Ongoing tutor and clinical laboratory assistant meetings provide opportunities for clinical faculty to clarify concepts and highlight any difficul-

ties their student group encountered. These sessions are in a variety of formats ranging from open discussions related to the learning scenarios being studied by the students, to more formal presentations of issues related to the evidence-based principles
of critical appraisal of the literature. Academic faculty often provide "mini-work-
shops" on EBP to clinical faculty. Clinical faculty have also been invited to attend
students' large group or seminar sessions. Several clinical faculty to participated in a
weekly interactive seminar course related to clinical measurement that occurred over
an eight-week period. The ongoing development of EBP skills has benefits for all
stakeholders. The clinical faculty member is able to participate in a professional development opportunity, the educational programs and the students benefit from the
faculty member's increased ability to facilitate and reinforce the students' EBP skills,
and the clinical facility has a clinician who is better able to implement EBP in the practice environment.

Assuming the role of facilitator in a student-centered curriculum provides an opportunity to develop new skills, many of which are transferable to the clinical setting.
Senior PT students who participated in a peer tutoring program (see Chapter 9) identified skills which would be relevant to clinical practice developed during their tutoring experience (Solomon and Crowe 1999). Analyses of the reflective journals kept
throughout their experience found that the students learned to ask more appropriate,
well-structured questions that they felt would assist in communicating with their clients. These students also reflected on the usefulness of the tutoring skills in assisting
in a number of educational roles they would be assuming in practice. Students recognized the value of developing group process skills and the usefulness of these skills
when interacting with health care teams and in staff meetings, when chairing a meeting, or when working on a research team. The skills identified by the peer tutors would
be of value to all health care practitioners and is another benefit of the clinical faculty
appointment identified by the clinical community.

Other tangible benefits include access to continuing education workshops and to
the library facilities. Clinical faculty have complimentary access to faculty development workshops related to educational roles and to special educational initiatives developed by the School of Rehabilitation Science. In the early to mid 1990s, access to an
email address and account was perceived as a major benefit by the clinical faculty. Currently, personal email is widely subscribed to and this is no longer viewed as a major
benefit. However, with the advent of electronic journals, faculty privileges allowing access to these are highly valued. Clinical faculty are also eligible for travel awards to
support presentations at conferences and for internal research competitions. Through
their part-time appointments, clinical faculty have links with the School of Rehabilitation Science research groups and projects and are invited to attend monthly meetings
and rounds.

There are other, less overt benefits. The concept of mentoring is incorporated in the
notion of community partnerships. Academic faculty often recognize the potential of
a clinician and encourage him or her to pursue opportunities that will enrich their career; this may be through approaching individuals to apply for a clinical faculty appointment, inviting a clinical faculty member to participate in a specific educational
or scholarly opportunity, or to enroll in an advanced degree.

And finally there are benefits to employees that go beyond providing staff with access to new information and skill development. In the tutoring survey, Tremblay et al.
(2001) found that many clinicians had negotiated time to participate in the educational programs when they commenced their employment. Employers have found that allowing therapists to participate in the educational programs assists in recruitment.

With the advent of innovative organizational structures, many clinicians have been placed in circumstances where their involvement in educational endeavors has been curtailed. As these organizational models become more mature, the hierarchical relationships within them are becoming clearer and the need for structures to support health professionals in remaining current in their practice and engaged with new learners has become evident. The clinical faculty appointments are a source for continuing professional development of the clinicians. Through ensuring an informed, involved, and energetic body of clinicians, employers can also ensure a happier, more productive workplace thus investing in retention as well as recruitment.

Other Community–University Initiatives

There are a number of other initiatives which have been of mutual benefit. These opportunities link areas of interest and focus on research, EBP, fieldwork placements, and the development of patient education materials.

Joint Research and Evidence-based Practice Initiatives

In an entry-level masters program, there is a delicate balance involved in the level of knowledge and skill that is transmitted concerning research skills and understanding. While we are not preparing students for research careers, we want to ensure they are skilled in the interpretation of evidence and familiar with research and program evaluation methods (see Chapter 5). Through the development of independent evidence-practice projects, the students work in partnership with clinicians to engage in a research process that links with the real world of practice. These clinician–student relationships come in a variety of forms. During the independent projects, clinicians are approached to define practice questions that are intriguing or of concern, and are offered the chance to participate with students in developing and undertaking a project that will be of value to their practice setting. Similarly, during the evidence-based small group seminars within the OT Program, clinicians are invited to pose a practice dilemma for the students to consider (see Chapter 5 for additional detail). The students search the literature to determine the "best practice" response to the dilemma, develop a mini-monograph, present it to their small group as an evaluated assignment and then provide the results to the clinician who posed the question. This particular initiative has produced excellent results in terms of reinforcing existing relationships and forging new ones. Throughout the evidence-based process within the curricula, the importance of relationships between faculty and clinician is highlighted. Faculty provide input to practice environments to enhance understanding of research principles and methods and engage in their own research on site. This last example serves to inculcate even closer relationships between these two professional spheres.

Emerging Roles Fieldwork Placements

The development of creative fieldwork placements in which students are placed in emergent areas of practice also has benefits for all stakeholders. The university is provided with new clinical fieldwork opportunities, which are often in short supply. Students develop consultation, marketing, and advocacy skills. Clinical facilities are pro-

Evidence-based Admissions in Rehabilitation Science

11

Penny Salvatori

In the late 1980s, a decision was made to phase out the Occupational Therapy (OT) and Physiotherapy (PT) Diploma Programs at Mohawk College in Hamilton, Ontario and develop two new second-degree baccalaureate programs at McMaster University. The curriculum design for the two new programs was based on the pedagogical principles of problem-based, self-directed, small group learning. Evidence-based practice was also a strong thread in terms of curriculum content. When a joint Occupational Therapy/Physiotherapy Admissions Committee was established in 1989, it was not surprising that a commitment was made to select candidates for the new problem-based learning programs using an evidence-based approach. Selecting the "best" candidates was important for several reasons: (1) there are always more qualified applicants than enrolment quotas allow, (2) it is essential to maximize enrolment and minimize student withdrawal, (3) it is important to maintain high standards of student performance, and (4) it is important that students' learning styles are congruent with the programs' educational philosophy and learning methods.

Using an evidence-based approach meant that decisions related to admission policy and procedures would be based on research and would entail the use of selection tools that demonstrate good psychometric properties and are cost-effective in terms of the time and resources required.

A Theoretical Framework for Student Selection

French and Rezler (1976) were the first to present a model for rational decision making in relation to student selection in the allied health professions. Dietrich (1981) adapted this framework by adding practical suggestions to instill greater objectivity in each of the four phases proposed by French and Rezler. We found this framework useful to guide our thinking and decision making in the initial stages of defining admission criteria and selecting screening tools.

Phase One

Phase one involves refining the criteria on which applicants should be evaluated. Desired characteristics and perceptible behaviors that the ideal candidate should display are defined. At McMaster University, the Admissions Committee identified the following basic characteristics as important for success in the programs and in the professions: intellectual ability, interpersonal skills, group skills, leadership qualities, written and oral communication skills, motivation, commitment, and past experience with people who are ill or disabled.

Phase Two

Phase two of the Dietrich framework involves selecting information sources where data can be quantified. These information tools should be selected on the basis of their reliability, validity, and generalizability. A literature review at the time indicated that academic grades and achievement tests were generally accepted as reliable and valid measures of intellectual ability and were the best predictors of success (Balogun et al. 1986; Bridle 1987; Higgs 1984; Oliver 1985; Schmalz et al. 1990; Sharp 1984; Tompkins and Harkins 1990). While there was good evidence to support the use of pre-admission academic grades in the selection process, there was little agreement in the literature regarding the use of additional screening measures. As Boyd et al. (1983 p. 182) suggested: "if professional schools are to succeed in their desire to increase heterogeneity of classes, eliminate the practitioners with poor interpersonal skills or those who will eventually abandon the profession, the solution will not be found in the continued use of traditional (academic) measures as the only determinants in the selection of potentially successful students." Selecting students for our non-traditional problem-based learning program added an additional challenge since the applicants' learning style and background experiences were of particular interest. Although a considerable body of research on traditional curricula supported the use of academic grades as predictors of performance, the Occupational Therapy/Physiotherapy Admissions Committee members were not convinced that these studies generalized well to the new small group learning, problem-based programs. Indeed, the few studies of such programs suggested that the predictive value of previous academic performance was less than substantial (Powis et al. 1988; Woodward and MacAuley 1983). Given the lack of convincing evidence that academic grades predicted subsequent performance in problem-based curricula, the Committee opted to use previous university grades only to establish eligibility for admission.

Following a review of the literature regarding other screening tools, the Committee decided to use a personal interview as the final stage of the admissions process, and to use a written submission to screen and rank applicants for interview. At that time there were numerous health science education programs using a personal interview in the selection process to assess non-cognitive characteristics such as empathy, self-confidence, communication skills, and interpersonal relationships. It was clear that reliability of the interview was improved when a structured format was used (Boyd et al. 1983; Powis et al. 1988; Richards et al. 1988) and when interviewers received prior training (Edwards et al. 1990; Heale et al. 1989). However, the question of predictive validity remained controversial, with some studies reporting a link between interview scores and student performance while others did not (Balogun et al. 1988; Graham and Boyd 1982; Heale et al. 1989; Levine et al. 1986; Posthuma and Sommerfreund 1985; Powis et al. 1988; Richards et al. 1988; Vojir and Bronstein 1983; Walker et al. 1985).

In our search for an appropriate written measure to screen applicants for interview, we reviewed several tools including the Kolb Learning Style Inventory, the Watson-Glazer Critical Thinking Scale, and the Self-Directed Learning Readiness Scale; however, all were discarded because of poor psychometric properties. Although there was a paucity of research on the use of written measures for student selection, four studies claimed that an "essay" was predictive of student performance (Balogun et al. 1986; Berchulc et al. 1987; Heale et al. 1989; Roehrig 1990). Dietrich (1981) suggested a written submission could be used to assess an applicant's affective domain as well as written communication skills. Hence, the decision was made to develop a new written submission tool for occupational therapy and physiotherapy applicants.

In summary, given the list (outlined above) of cognitive and non-cognitive characteristics considered important for assessment of candidates, the Admissions Committee decided on a three-stage admission process using:

- Pre-admission grades as an indicator of intellectual ability to establish basic eligibility for admission

- A written autobiographical submission (ABS) to assess the applicants' knowledge of the profession and the McMaster program, as well as their motivation and related experience, and also to screen applicants for interview

■ A personal interview using a structured format to assess interpersonal skills, communication abilities, and self-assessment skills

This three-stage admission process remained in place with some modifications for the first 14 years of our 15-year history.

Phase Three

Phase three of the Dietrich framework consists of transforming data from information sources into measurable forms. The Committee developed rating scales and objective scoring criteria for three separate selection tools (the two-part ABS and the personal interview) in an effort to quantify the attributes of interest and to measure the extent to which the applicant possessed those attributes. Volunteer assessors were recruited from among faculty, community health professionals, alumni, and current students. They were asked to read and score the applicants' sketches and letters, and/or interview candidates. To enhance standardization of the process and maximize reliability, all volunteers were required to attend training sessions.

Phase Four

The final, yet likely most important, phase is evaluation. Dietrich (1981) suggests that an iterative process to assess the reliability and validity of admissions criteria and procedures acts as an internal control mechanism and provides for public accountability. From the very beginning, since the first intake of students in the fall of 1990, the Admissions Committee was committed to evidence-based decision making. Since reliability is a necessary but not sufficient condition of validity (Nunnally 1970), initial research and development efforts were devoted to designing and investigating the reliability of the selection tools. Predictive validity using in-course academic and clinical grades as the outcomes of interest was the focus of our research in later years. The limitation of using only in-course grades as the outcome of interest is recognized. Long-term follow-up studies to explore other outcomes of interest such as competence in practice, leadership roles, and career profiles were not considered feasible at that time. Fifteen years of research has resulted in many modifications and changes to the admissions policy and selection procedures. Certain tools have been discarded, some have been redesigned, some new tools have been developed, and various weightings have been changed over the years in terms of determining final offers of admission. Figures 11.1 and 11.2 provide an overview of the admission process used in the BHSc (Occupational Therapy) and BHSc (Physiotherapy) Programs from 1990 to 1999 and currently in the MSc (Occupational Therapy) and MSc (Physiotherapy) Programs.

Pre-admission Academic Grades

In the BHSc program, once an applicant established his or her eligibility for admission, the grade point average (GPA) was not looked at again, thereby giving no advantage to applicants with higher grades. The GPA requirements at McMaster University were different from other rehabilitation programs. Some applicants, especially those without a science background or with a lower overall GPA, were able to be competitive with other students and meet the admission requirements.

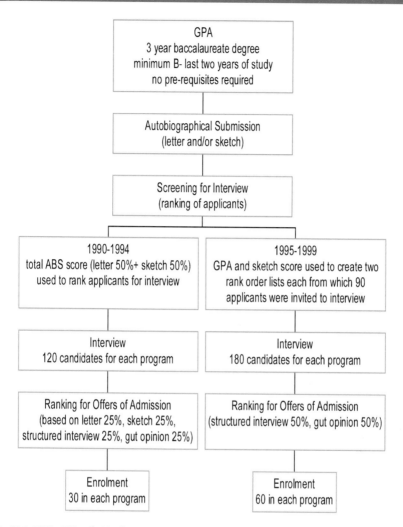

Fig. 11.1. BHSc OT and PT admissions process 1990–1999

Findings from our first predictive validity study (1995) clearly identified pre-admission GPA as the best predictor of in-course performance in both the Occupational Therapy and Physiotherapy Programs, whether measured as year 1 GPA, year 2 GPA, or overall graduation GPA (year 1 + year 2). Pearson correlation coefficients ranged from .29 to .37 and the relationship was statistically significant. A policy decision was made to begin to use GPA to a greater extent than to simply establish a candidate's eligibility. As of fall 1995, all applicants were ranked for interview on the basis of both pre-admission GPA and their written ABS score. The list of 180 interviewees for each program was compiled by drawing the top 90 candidates off each list. This meant that an applicant with a high ABS score but low GPA or an applicant who ranked high on the GPA list but low on the ABS list could be invited for an interview.

Ongoing predictive validity analyses confirmed that GPA was still the best predictor of in-course performance in both BHSc programs. This finding is consistent with

Fig. 11.2. MSc OT and PT admissions process 2004

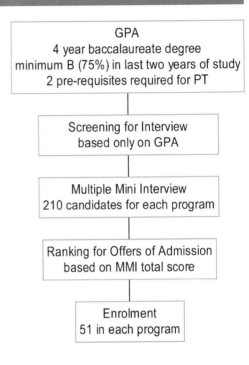

Table 11.1. The use of pre-admission GPA in the MSc programs

Year	GPA required[a]	Number of applicants	Number offered interviews	GPA cut-off for interview	Purpose of GPA
2000 (first class)	3.0/4.0 (or B)	OT 207 PT 516	150 150	3.12 3.65	Used to establish eligibility and rank 50% of candidates for interview
2001	As above	OT 258 PT 619	As above	3.30 3.72	As above
2002	As above	OT 368 PT 851	As above	3.27 3.63	As above
2003	As above	OT 370 PT 850	180 180	3.27 3.62	Used to establish eligibility and rank 100% of candidates for interview
2004	As above	OT 475 PT 890	210 210	3.36 3.62	As above

[a] Additional prerequisites were required of MSc(PT) applicants

the health sciences literature (Salvatori 2001). In 2000, as new admissions policies and procedures were being put in place for the first applicants to the new masters-level Occupational Therapy and Physiotherapy Programs, consistent evidence of a strong correlation between pre-admission GPA and in-course performance could no longer be ignored. As a result, in addition to requiring a completed four-year honors degree (or equivalent), the minimum GPA requirement was increased to a B (or 3.0/4.0 or 75 percent) in the last two years of full-time study. For physiotherapy applicants only, two prerequisite courses were also required: a half or full credit course with a B average in both a biological or life science and a social science or humanities course.

In 2003, a decision was made to use pre-admission GPA alone to rank applicants for interview. Table 11.1 illustrates the use of the pre-admission GPA over the first four years of the MSc Occupational Therapy and Physiotherapy Programs. The GPA cut-off for interview has been relatively stable during this period for both programs, although slightly lower overall as compared to latter years of the BHSc Programs.

Autobiographical Submission

The written ABS used in the second stage of the selection process changed over time from an eight-page two-part submission, to a much shorter three-page one-part submission, to being eliminated completely as a measure to screen applicants for interview. Initially, the Admissions Committee decided to use the ABS as the sole screening measure to rank applicants for interview. To establish face validity and content validity, committee members debated the qualities that best characterized the successful occupational therapy and physiotherapy student and practitioner. This consensus exercise resulted in a two-part ABS to be completed by all candidates. Part one, the letter of application, was a two-page essay-type written paper that was assessed using a seven-point scale in four categories: (1) knowledge of the occupational therapy or physiotherapy profession, (2) knowledge of the unique features of the Occupational Therapy or Physiotherapy Program, (3) self-assessment abilities in terms of personal fit and motivation, and (4) writing skills.

Part two, the point-form autobiographical sketch, originally consisted of six categories: (1) work experiences, (2) learning experiences, (3) leadership experiences, (4) teamwork experiences, (5) experiences which demonstrate curiosity and creativity, and (6) experiences which have influenced personal attitudes toward illness and disability. Applicants were required to list their experiences within each category and demonstrate insight by outlining the relevance of their experiences to the study and practice of occupational therapy or physiotherapy. Assessor guidelines were developed using a seven-point rating scale for each category. Both the letter of application and sketch were read and scored independently by three assessors.

Assessors for the ABS were drawn from the faculty, clinical community, and student body. A mandatory three-hour training session provided an overview of the Programs, a review of the admissions process, and a description of the assessor's role and responsibilities. Using simulated sketches and letters prepared by the Committee, assessors then practiced using the rating guidelines and scoring applicants. Scores were compared and discussed in terms of expectations of applicants and overall rater agreement. Assessors were instructed to read the sketches and letters independently, scoring one at a time, and not to discuss their assessments with others. Assessors provided valuable feedback related to the need for clarifying instructions to applicants, improving the rating criteria and scale descriptors for the assessors, and providing more examples of applicants' responses in the training session. For the first five admissions cycles (1990–1994), the letter and sketch were weighted 25 percent each in the final ranking for offers of admission.

From 1991 to 1993, three more consensus exercises involving community clinicians were conducted in attempts to improve inter-rater reliability of the sketch for the work experience, leadership, and teamwork categories. Rating guidelines and rating scales were revised and more examples were provided for practice purposes at the training sessions. Table 11.2 provides an example of the revisions made to the work experience category. Assessors were now instructed to score the ABS packages across applicants within categories in order to promote more consistent scoring and minimize any within-applicant "halo-effect."

Reliability analysis conducted over the first six years of the BHSc Programs indicated a steady improvement in reliability of both the letter of application and the autobiographical sketch (see Table 11.3). Gains in reliability were linked to more detailed instructions to applicants, example-supported rating guidelines, increased rater practice during training sessions, and increased rater experience. A generalizability analysis conducted in 1993 showed that the six sketch categories could be reduced to three without significant loss of reliability. An additional study based on rater type revealed no systematic differences among faculty, community, and student ratings which meant it was possible to use mixed rater groups without increasing an inherent bias. This was welcome news from a resource perspective since the faculty group was the smallest in number.

The predictive validity analysis for the sketch and letter (1995) revealed less positive findings. Pearson correlation coefficients between letter scores and in-course performance ranged from –.23 to +.27 for physiotherapy students and –.37 to +.15 for occupational therapy students. These correlations were poor and the numerous negative correlations were disturbing, suggesting that the scores some applicants received on their letter of application were inversely correlated with their performance as students in the programs. The predictive validity of the sketch was marginally better with a similar range of correlations (–.27 to +.23 for physiotherapy students; –.25 to +.22 for occupational therapy students); however, there were many more positive correlations overall. In addition, results indicated a significant correlation between the sketch scores and the Inquiry Seminar course grades for year 2 occupational therapy students ($.22, P=.05$) and year 1 physiotherapy students ($.30, P=.000$).

In 1995, given the increasing number of applications to both programs, the corresponding increase in the number of volunteer assessors required to score the ABSs, and the poor predictive validity of the letter, the decision was made to discontinue the letter and rank applicants for interviews using a shortened three-category sketch. Although the predictive validity of the sketch was not good, it was better than the letter and there was no existing reliable and valid tool that could screen applicants for interview. The sketch categories of work, learning, and teamwork experiences were retained because of their overall superior reliability.

In 2001, the second predictive validity study revealed improvement in the correlation of sketch scores and in-course performance with Pearson coefficients ranging from –.21 to +.82 for physiotherapy students and –.20 to +.42 for occupational therapy students; however, overall mean correlations remained low. Salvatori (2001) has discussed the ongoing controversy related to the reliability and validity of written submissions used in the selection of students for the health professions. The Admissions Committee was concerned that the ABS assessment process was very resource-intensive and also that some applicants were not submitting their own written material.

Table 11.2. Rating guidelines for work experience category (1990–1991). Minimum score = 0, maximum score = 7. Assign 0 to applicants who fail to attain the minimum requirement for a score of 1. In addition, for insight: −1, 0, +1

Without a health focus			With a health focus			
Unrelated to OT/PT	Minimally related to OT/PT (person/people focus)		Moderately related to OT/PT		Significantly related to OT/PT	
	Casual unstructured contact	Sustained contact	Fitness/activity related or limited contact with ill/disabled populations		Sustained/structured contact with ill/disabled populations	
Cashier Laborer Clerk	Waitress Library worker Hospital worker (kitchen, housekeeping) Secretary/ receptionist Business Owner/operator	Teacher/ instructor Coach Massage therapist assistant	CPR instructor Research assistant in gait laboratory	Hospital worker Volunteer porter Masseur/ masseuse Fitness appraiser Nursing aide Mental health counselor	Non-OT/PT setting Nurse Kinesiologist Exercise physiologist Activation therapist	OT/PT setting OT/PT aide Hydrotherapist
1	2	3	4	5	6	7

Table 11.3. Overall reliability of the autobiographical submission. Reliability is measured by the intraclass correlation coefficient

	1990		1994		1996	
	OT	PT	OT	PT	OT	PT
Autobiographical sketch	.32	.21	.88	.87	.79	.77
Letter of application	.46	.16	.83	.83	n/a	n/a

In stark contrast to the ABS results, our research findings reconfirmed the superior predictive validity of the pre-admission GPA. As a result, the Committee voted unanimously to eliminate the autobiographical sketch as a screening tool and bring applicants to interview solely on the basis of pre-admission GPA. This new policy was implemented during the 2003 admission cycle.

Personal Interview

The personal interview has served as the final stage of the admission process for the past 15 years, and the sole basis for ranking candidates for offers of admission for the last 10 years. It has been used to assess those non-cognitive personal qualities deemed important for success in the program and as future health care professionals. The format has consistently embraced a structured, standardized approach versus an open-ended interview; however, it has been modified over time from a single panel interview to three separate individual interviews to a seven-station multiple mini-interview.

The initial development of the interview tool followed a framework described by Streiner and Norman (1989): (1) devising items, (2) scaling responses, (3) selecting items, (4) scoring responses, (5) controlling bias, and (6) pilot testing. Initially items for the interview tool were derived from consultation with McMaster faculty, the review of philosophy and scopes of practice documents for the professions, and the health sciences literature. As reliability improved with the use of a structured format and trained interviewers, the Admissions Committee condensed the items into a 30-minute structured interview to assess the following: motivation, ability to relate, adaptability/flexibility, ability to evaluate self and others, maturity, ethical principles, and communication skills.

A final category of "overall opinion" was added. The bank of questions that was developed by the Canadian Dental Association (CDA) served as the major source of questions to address the above domains of interest. As outlined by Boyd et al. (1983), the CDA structured interview questions were developed to be clearly understood, not require inferential judgments, minimize rater bias, be open-ended to avoid a yes/no response, meet legal standards, and not require a "right" or socially desirable answer.

The next step was to decide how the interviewers would rate or score each applicant's responses to the questions. A continuous response scale was selected over a categorical yes/no response scale since it would provide more valuable and precise information on the applicant and should improve overall reliability. The interviewer would be requested to provide a direct quantitative estimate of the magnitude of the attribute being assessed. A modified seven-point Likert scale was chosen because of its easy design and administration and its potential range of scores. According to Streiner and Norman (1989 p. 27), the "minimum number of categories used by raters should be in the region of 5 to 7." An odd number of rating points was purposely chosen to give the interviewer the option of a neutral position along the scale.

To ensure fairness and control for interviewer bias, it was decided that each applicant would be interviewed by a panel of three drawn from the faculty, community clinicians, and students. Attempts were made to control for additional sources of bias in order to reduce variance among interviewers and thus improve overall reliability. For example, to reduce social desirability bias, applicants were told that there are no "right" or "wrong" answers. To reduce end-aversion bias and improve the discriminatory power of the scale, the interviewers were trained to use the entire range of scores on the scale. To reduce a possible halo effect, subjectivity, and any value-laden attitudinal bias, the interviewers did not have any prior knowledge of the applicant such as access to the academic record or ABS score. All assessors were trained to rate responses to the interview questions on the basis of evidence provided by the applicant rather than on a global impression. Each interviewer rated independently of the other raters on the team, and no discussion or alteration of final scores was allowed. A small pilot test of the new interview tool was conducted before the process was adopted.

Ninety interviewers were recruited for the first round of selection interviews and were required to attend a five-hour training session. The videotapes from the pilot testing served to illustrate the standardized format and provide examples of applicant responses. Participants were asked to rate the applicant responses (on video) to each of the 18 questions and these ratings were then used to promote group discussion. Some additional modification of the questions and guidelines followed at this point.

Interviews were conducted over a two-week period. Each team interviewed six applicants in a half-day session. Interviewers were instructed to rate each applicant independently and were blinded to the scores of other interviewers on the team. The total 18-item interview score and the overall opinion score were combined with the applicant's sketch and letter scores (each weighted 25 percent) to yield a final admission score. These scores were used to rank applicants and select 30 students for each of the new Occupational Therapy and Physiotherapy Programs.

Since the implementation of the structured interview in 1990, feedback was sought annually from interviewers and interviewees. In addition, a research program was put in place to explore the reliability and validity of the new interview tool. Changes for the 1992 admissions cycle included the following minor revisions: eliminating category titles, for example, motivation, ability to relate; rewording specific questions; inserting statements to precede the questions to improve the natural conversational flow; and intensifying interviewer training to improve the raters' confidence in using the scoring criteria.

The first study conducted in 1990 entailed the use of four simulated applicants. The simulated applicants were trained to provide a spectrum of responses to the standardized interview questions. The simulated applicants were interspersed with the real applicants during interview week. Each simulated applicant was interviewed by each of four teams. Generalizability analysis revealed a significant "team effect" and further suggested that interview teams could be reduced in size from three to two interviewers without any significant loss of reliability. Despite the independent review process, it was clear that a team effect was influencing the interviewers' scores. Results also showed, however, that there were no systematic differences across ratings from faculty, community clinicians, or student interviewers. As a result, in 1992 through to 1994, each applicant was interviewed by two interview teams (three-rater teams in 1992 and 1993; two-rater teams in 1994). The total set of 18 interview questions were divided across teams of interviewers in an attempt to minimize a potential team effect, to disperse the halo effect, and to enhance the fairness of the process. As a result of further analysis, as of 1995, every applicant was interviewed separately by three individuals, making the best use of available resources and available research evidence. See Fig. 11.3 for sample interview questions and scoring criteria.

A reliability analysis of the occupational therapy admissions process after the first two admission cycles (Salvatori et al. 1992) revealed intraclass correlation coefficients (ICCs) of .72 to .75 for the structured set of questions and .76 to .77 for the overall opinion score. The internal consistency was .94. These preliminary findings were encouraging and demonstrated that reliability was acceptable. Subsequent reliability studies revealed much variability from year to year with ICCs ranging from a low of .45 to a high of .93. It is possible that the lower reliability coefficients were the result of a "restricted range" problem, i.e., a more narrow range of interview scores, reflecting a more homogeneous group of applicants and increased difficulty to discriminate among applicants.

LITTLE EVIDENCE		SOME EVIDENCE		GOOD EVIDENCE		STRONG EVIDENCE	
1	2	3	4	5	6	7	

a) **As a result of the rapid changes occurring in health care, what are the current issues facing the profession of Occupational Therapy?**

Look for evidence of knowledge of current issues facing the professions (**e.g.** decreasing government funding, trend to community health care, new models of service delivery, privatization of health care, increase in aging and disabled populations, high technology, need for outcome-based/effectiveness research, consumerism movement, public accountability, self-regulation, private practice issues, new emerging roles).

In determining your score, consider the applicant's breadth of knowledge of the profession beyond day-to-day clinical practice.

b) **Functioning as a team member is an essential element of this programme. What qualities and skills do you possess that will help you support your peers and also contribute to their learning?**

Look for evidence of a willingness to participate in a supportive learning environment and insight into personal strengths which may enhance the learning of other students (e.g. empathy, listening skills, patience, flexibility to balance personal and group goals, academic background, life experiences).

c) **If you were offered admission to the Occupational Therapy Programme, what do you see as the challenges that lie ahead of you and how do you plan to meet them?**

Look for evidence of insight into his/her ability to meet the requirements of the programme (e.g. ability to adapt to a new way of learning, pace and workload of the Programme, family responsibilities, age, finances, new to student role, disability, travel requirements/commuting, out-of-town placements).

Overall Opinion

UNSUITABLE		BORDERLINE		SUITABLE		OUTSTANDING	
1	2	3	4	5	6	7	

Use the above scale to provide a rating of your overall opinion regarding the suitability of the applicant. In formulating your opinion, consider whether this person is someone you would like to teach (if you are a faculty member), or work with (if you are a clinician) or study with (if you are a student).

Fig. 11.3. Sample interview questions and rating guidelines

The predictive validity study for the first five cohorts of students suggested a positive relationship between the structured interview score and in-course GPA for both physiotherapy and occupational therapy students. Correlations ranged from .29 (P=.02) to .39 (P<.05) for the physiotherapy students, and from .27 (P<.05) to .38 (P<.04) for the occupational therapy students. In addition, for the occupational therapy students, there was a positive correlation between the overall gut opinion interview score and GPA with correlations ranging from .26, P=.05 to .44, P<.02. The results of this predictive validity study served to validate the continued use of the interview in the selection process. Given the interview was a stronger predictor of student performance than the ABS, a decision was made to continue to use pre-admission GPA to establish eligibility, use the autobiographical sketch to screen for interview, and use only the interview score (with equal weighting of the structured interview score and gut opinion score) for final ranking of applicants for offers of admission.

For the first three admission cycles of the new masters entry-level programs, the admission process remained the same, i.e., using pre-admission GPA and sketch score to rank applicants for interview and using interview scores alone to rank candidates for offers of admission. However, the Admissions Committee remained concerned that the interview questions were common knowledge, that some pre-interview training was occurring behind the scenes, and that the autobiographical sketch was not always the applicant's own work. For the 2003 admission cycle, a decision was made to eliminate the sketch, to screen applicants for interview using pre-admission GPA only, and to increase the number of applicants interviewed.

At the same time, colleagues in the MD Program at McMaster University were in the process of developing and pilot testing a new interview format referred to as the Multiple Mini-Interview (MMI). The MMI is similar to the Objective Structured Clinical Examination (OSCE) commonly used to assess students' clinical skills in health sciences programs (Eva et al. 2004b). The MMI involves a series of interview stations through which the applicants rotate. Each station is ten minutes in duration with two minutes allowed for the applicant to read the question or scenario posted outside the interview door followed by eight minutes for the applicant to answer the interviewer's questions inside the interview room. A bell sounds at two and eight minutes to keep the candidates moving. Since the MMI involves multiple ratings of each applicant from multiple raters, it is considered to be fair and reliable.

In 2003, the MMI was pilot tested using a short three-station interview circuit, 77 occupational therapy and physiotherapy volunteer applicants as study subjects, and 30 interviewers (two per station) drawn from the faculty, clinical community, and student body. Analysis of results revealed good internal consistency, inter-rater reliability, and discriminant validity. Interstation correlations were low indicating the need for more stations. Using generalizability analysis, the overall reliability co-efficient of a three-station circuit and two interviewers per station was .51 (as compared to .39 for the structured interview). The reliability could be improved to .68 (for a six-station circuit, and two interviewers per station) or to .77 (for a 12-station circuit and one interviewer per station). Feedback from applicants and interviewers was also very positive. As a result of this small pilot study, as well as validity testing in the MD Program (Eva et al. 2004a), the Admissions Committee decided to replace the structured interview with the MMI. Resources in terms of potential interviewers and room availability naturally limited the size of the MMI that could be developed. Accordingly, the decision was made to use a seven-station MMI and one interviewer per station. The new MMI format allowed us to combine the benefits of our previous interview process (with structured questions and standardized rating criteria) with the special features of the MMI which included probing the applicant's responses and assessing the applicant's ability to analyze ethical scenarios.

In 2004, the new MMI was implemented. Approximately 420 applicants were interviewed. The MMI involved seven interview stations for each applicant over a 70-minute period. Each of the seven stations had a different focus. Four of the stations pursued the applicant's knowledge of: (1) the occupational therapy or physiotherapy profession, (2) the McMaster Occupational Therapy or Physiotherapy Program, (3) problem-based learning, and (4) health care issues in general. Three of the stations involved ethical scenarios that required moral reasoning. Interviewers were drawn from the faculty, clinical community, and student body and were required to attend a training session. Applicants were assessed at each MMI station on the quality of his/her response, general communication skills, and overall impression in terms of suitability for the McMaster program and/or profession. Overall reliability was .70 for the occupational therapy interviews and .68 for the physiotherapy interviews. These results suggest a remarkable improvement in reliability as compared to data on the structured interview. The Admissions Committee was pleased with these results and remains committed to the use of the MMI in the future; see Fig. 11.2 for an overview of the current admission process. Future studies will entail ongoing reliability assessment of the MMI and validity testing in terms of in-course performance of occupational therapy and physiotherapy students.

Lessons Learned

Over the past 15 years, we have learned much about using theory and expert opinion to guide the development of admission tools, and using research evidence to improve the reliability, validity, and efficiency of the admissions process. The importance of using selection tools congruent with our problem-based learning curricula also had a significant impact on our decision making. The theoretical framework described by Dietrich (1981) proved useful in developing an overall development plan and in selecting screening tools. The measurement framework outlined by Streiner and Norman (1989) also proved useful as a guide to develop, implement, and evaluate the use of a personal interview in the selection process.

Research, either reported in the health sciences literature or generated internally, has guided all decision making of the Admissions Committee since its inception in 1989. As a result, an evidence-based admissions process has evolved over time. As Youdas et al. (1992) have suggested, and we have confirmed through our own experience, reliability can be improved with clearer assessor guidelines, specific rating criteria, anchored rating scales, training of assessors, and use of experienced assessors. Although reliability can be improved and remain relatively stable over time, it is clear that yearly fluctuations will occur. This means that a longitudinal evaluation process should be put in place in order to avoid hasty decisions. While we made minor changes to the admissions procedures on an annual basis, the major changes in admissions policy occurred at four- or five-year intervals.

It is also clear that as the number of applicants increased over time, homogeneity of the top-ranked candidates also increased. For example, the background education and the pre-admission GPAs became increasingly similar. This was particularly true of physiotherapy candidates whose sheer numbers raised the cut-off pre-admission GPA for eligibility and whose background is predominately in science, often kinesiology. Higher pre-admission GPAs create a "restriction of range" problem which, in turn, means it is more difficult to discriminate among applicants, thus resulting in lower reliability coefficients. Higher in-course GPAs result in a similar problem resulting in lower validity coefficients. As Elam and Andrynowski (1991) have suggested, it is important to be more accepting of lower reliability and validity coefficients, particularly in a multifactorial admissions process such as ours, since they may indeed be stronger than they first appear.

Furthermore, as Nunnally (1970) has suggested, reliability is a necessary but not sufficient condition for validity. We have shown that a reliable student selection tool (such as the autobiographical letter and sketch) is not necessarily predictive of in-course performance. This means overall that evaluation of the admissions process is very complicated, should be ongoing, and necessitates several years of research. It should also be pointed out that our predictive validity studies included only those applicants who were admitted, leaving unanswered the question of whether those not admitted would have performed equally as well. Given that the validity coefficients range from .30 to .40, only about 10 to 15 percent of the variance in student in-course grades can be accounted for in terms of admission scores. Further research is needed to identify other factors that contribute to student success.

In general, we learned to be open-minded and embrace an experimental process. We were not only committed to using theory and research to make decisions but also declared our openness to feedback and suggestions from key stakeholders along the way.

Conclusions

The 15-year evolution of an evidence-based decision-making process to establish admission policy and procedures for selecting students to the Occupational Therapy and Physiotherapy Programs at McMaster University has been described. We have based all decisions on the principles of theory, research, and cost-efficiency. The low program attrition rate and the success of our graduates in practice would appear to attest to the overall success of the admissions process.

Our research has clearly shown that pre-admission GPA is the best predictor of in-course performance in both the Occupational Therapy and Physiotherapy Programs. This is an important finding since the Admissions Committee was not convinced initially that this relationship would hold true for students in a problem-based learning program. Pre-admission GPA is now the sole screening tool used to rank applicants for interview. Although the autobiographical written submission was found to be a reliable measure in terms of discriminating among applicants, its predictive validity was poor and, as a result, both components were eliminated as screening measures. The structured interview tool was found to be reliable and demonstrate acceptable validity. The new MMI interview used for admission to the masters entry-level programs shows much promise as a reliable measure to assess personal attributes such as interpersonal/communication skills, self-assessment abilities, and moral reasoning skills; however, validity has yet to be determined. As Salvatori (2001) concluded, ongoing research is needed to find more reliable and valid ways of assessing the non-cognitive characteristics of applicants, particularly in the context of actual performance in practice. Since admissions scores only account for minimal variance in in-course performance, other factors contributing to student success need to be explored.

The changes we have made over the last 15 years have resulted in a more efficient and cost-effective process. The Admissions Committee remains committed to an evidence-based admissions process. Our research efforts will continue as will our commitment to increase both the gender mix (aimed at admitting more males in the Occupational Therapy Program) and ethnic mix of the student body (including aboriginal Canadians and international students). Admissions Committees in other rehabilitation science programs are encouraged to use our experiences to guide their decisions in identifying appropriate admission criteria, selecting measures to assess both the cognitive and non-cognitive attributes of applicants, weighing various factors in the final ranking of candidates, and evaluating the overall admissions process.

References

Balogun JA, Karacoloff LA, Farina NT (1986) Predictors of academic achievement in physical therapy. Phys Ther 66:976–980

Berchulc CM, Wade GA, Seider KK (1987) Predicting academic achievement of undergraduate occupational therapy students: preliminary results. Occup Ther J Res 7:245–248

Boyd MA, Graham JW, Teteruck WR, Krupka J (1983) Development and implementation of a structured interview for dental admissions. J Can Dent Assoc 3:181–185

Bridle MJ (1987) Student selection: a comparison of three methods. Can J Occup Ther 54:113–117

Dietrich M (1981) Putting objectivity in the allied health student selection process. J Allied Health 10:26–39

Edwards JC, Johnson EK, Molidor JB (1990) The interview in the admission process. Acad Med 65:167–177

Elam CL, Andrykowski MA (1991) Admission interview ratings: relationship to applicant academic and demographic variables and interviewer characteristics. Acad Med 66:S13–S15

Eva KW, Reiter HI, Rosenfeld J, Norman GR (2004a) The ability of the multiple mini-interview to predict pre-clerkship performance in medical school. Acad Med 79:S1–S3

Eva KW, Rosenfeld J, Reiter HI, Norman GR (2004b) An admission OSCE: the multiple mini-interview. Med Educ 38:314–326

French RM, Rezler AG (1976) Student selection in four-year programs. In: Ford CW, Gordon MK (eds) Teaching in the health professions. Mosby, St Louis, MI

Graham JW, Boyd MA (1982) A structured interview for dental school admissions. J Dent Educ 4:78–82

Heale JA, Blumberg P, Wakefield J, McAuley R (1989) The relationship between admission selection scores and performance of family medicine residents, McMaster University

Higgs ZR (1984) Predicting success in nursing: from prototype to pragmatics. West J Nurs Res 6:77–95

Levine SB, Knecht HG, Eisen RG (1986) Selection of physical therapy students: interview methods and academic predictors. J Allied Health 15:143–151

Nunnally JC (1970) Introduction to psychological measurement. McGraw-Hill, New York, NY

Oliver DH (1985) The relationship of selected admission criteria to the academic success of associate degree nursing students. J Nurs Educ 24:197–206

Posthuma BW, Sommerfreund J (1985) Examination of selection criteria for a program in occupational therapy. Am J Occup Ther 39:441–445

Powis DA, Neame RLB, Bristow T, Murphy LB (1988) The objective structured interview for medical student selection. Med Educ 296:765–768

Richards P, McManus IC, Maitlis SA (1988) Reliability of interviewing in medical student selection. Br Med J Clin Res 296:1520–1521

Roehrig S (1990) Prediction of student problems in a baccalaureate physical therapy program. J Phys Ther Educ 4:26–30

Salvatori P (2001) Reliability and validity of admissions tools used to select students for the health professions. Adv Health Sci Educ 6:159–175

Salvatori P, Heale H, Stratford P (1992) The development and reliability assessment of a structured interview for occupational therapy student selection. Paper presentation at the American Educational Research Association conference, San Francisco, 23 April 1992

Schmalz GM, Rahr RR, Allen RM (1990) The use of pre-admission data to predict levels of success in selected allied health students. Occup Ther J Res 10:367–376

Sharp TG (1984) An analysis of the relationship of seven selected variables to State Board test pool examination performance of the University of Tennessee, Knoxville, College of Nursing. J Nurs Educ 23:57–63

Streiner DL, Norman GR (1989) Health measurement scales. Oxford University Press, New York, NY

Tompkins LS, Harkins CJ (1990) Predicting academic success in a nontraditional program. J Allied Health 19:15–24

Vojir CP, Bronstein RA (1983) Applicant selection procedures: a more objective approach to the interview process. J Allied Health 12:95–102

Walker JD, Killip DE, Fuller JL (1985) The significance of the admission interview in predicting students' performance in dental school. J Med Educ 60:569–571

Woodward CA, McAuley RG (1983) Can the academic background of medical graduates be detected during internship? Can Med Assoc J 129:567–569

Youdas JW, Hallman HO, Carey JR, Bogard CL, Garrett TR (1992) Reliability and validity of judgments of applicant essays as a predictor of academic success in an entry-level physical therapy education program. J Phys Ther Educ 6:15–18

Educational Preparation for Rural and Remote Practice: The Northern Studies Stream

12

Jennifer Cano, Elaine Foster-Seargeant

Contents

Internationally there has been an increased interest in improving the quality of rural health and rural health care services. The Northern Health Information Partnership (2004) indicates that rural citizens and their communities have poorer measures of health status than their urban counterparts. Although the reasons for these differences are complex, there is widespread agreement regarding the lack of quality health care services for rural citizens. A significant component of this underservicing is attributed to the shortage of health care professionals (Humphreys et al. 2000; Strasser et al. 2000).

Rural communities focus on the recruitment and retention of heath care professionals in an attempt to remedy the shortage of health care providers. To be successful, new recruits need to develop unique rural practice skills. The majority of practicing rural health care providers do not have postgraduate education related to the challenges of rural practice and have difficulty accessing this training once they are practicing (Kenny and Ducket 2003). This challenge can be addressed by including training for rural practice in the professional education of health care providers.

This chapter presents an innovative program to train occupational therapists and physiotherapists for northern, rural, and remote practice. The primary focus of the Northern Studies Stream is to prepare occupational therapy and physiotherapy students from McMaster University for the challenges and rewards of rural practice. The reader will be introduced to the context in which Northern Ontario rehabilitation practitioners work and a program that endeavors to prepare clinicians for this practice. Insights gained over 14 years of program implementation and evaluation will be shared.

The Northern Studies Stream Program

In 1990, McMaster University recognized the importance of specific rural training and the need to improve recruitment of rehabilitation professionals to rural communities. A unique program, the Northern Studies Stream, was created to prepare occupational therapists and physiotherapists for rural practice. The Northern Studies Stream in Thunder Bay, Ontario, functions as a satellite campus of McMaster University. The program's main goal is to prepare students for practice in rural and northern areas, and encourage them to return to these sites after graduation.

The mandate of the Northern Studies Stream is:

- To increase students' awareness and knowledge of the determinants of health unique to northern and rural communities

- To increase students' awareness of First Nations' health concerns and practices

- To provide students with the skills required for the unique practice of rural health care

Over the course of the two-year program one half of the students enrolled in the Physiotherapy and Occupational Therapy Programs have a Northern Studies Stream experience. This takes the form of a combined eight-week academic unit followed by a six-week clinical placement or a clinical placement alone. After 14 years 600 students have participated in the Northern Studies Stream.

The provincial government funds this initiative by providing monies for students' travel and accommodation while in the north. The funding allows students to test attitudes and expectations of rural practice without undue financial hardship.

While there is consistency in the educational objectives between programs delivered in Hamilton and Thunder Bay, there is flexibility that permits the Northern Studies Stream to meet its mandate. For example, many of the case scenarios that drive the learning in the tutorial setting are based on clients from northern communities and address the unique socioeconomic and geographic realities of rural life. Although the problems are similar to those used by their counterparts at the main McMaster campus, Northern Studies Stream students are expected to place their client within a northern or rural community context. Students access information from local resources, agencies, and community experts to gather information about how to best meet the needs of their theoretical client. This search process teaches students to adapt their strategies for accessing the latest evidence to the resources available in rural communities, often relying more on web-based journals and texts. This strategy also highlights the unique methods of health care delivery in the north and the service provision variability between the north and south.

While the vast majority of teaching takes place onsite, technology in the form of videoconferencing is used to maintain communication with students at the McMaster campus and allow faculty from both campuses to teach classes simultaneously to both groups. In an effort to bridge the potential gap in accessing information caused by geographical isolation, Northern Studies Stream faculty and students have access to an information/library specialist who orients students to the reality of study and clinical practice in the north. Students are guided through strategies to access information from a distance. The same service is offered to the clinicians in Northwestern Ontario who have become skilled in staying current electronically. These clinicians are role models for students.

Students are also introduced to the many continuing professional development programs available in Northwestern Ontario through Health Sciences North. They are introduced to philosophies and practical strategies that may help them to thrive in a northern, rural, and remote community after graduation.

As the literature suggests that recreational and lifestyle opportunities are significant recruitment factors, students are also encouraged to explore the recreation possibilities available in the north (e.g., camping, skiing, theater, and dog sledding). Thus students are exposed to broad aspects of living in the north from both personal and professional perspectives.

The Context of Northern, Rural, and Remote Practice

Developing an understanding of the context in which northern, rural, and remote rehabilitation practice occurs is an important component of the students' learning. Some of the issues introduced to the students are common to other geographic areas that are northern or rural or remote, but very few locales can be described as combining all three. It is important for the students to understand the multiple layers of influence that this combination has on clinical practice.

What is Rural?

There are commonly described physical, social, institutional, and cultural characteristics of the term rural. One study described the rural practice environment as characterized by low population density, vulnerable and fragile organizations, and small populations with long travel distances to other communities and health care providers (Hart et al. 2002). Other characteristics of the rural practice environment have included geographical isolation (Bent 1999; Hegney and McCarthy 2000; Kohler and Mayberry 1993; Mills and Millsteed 2002), increased dependence on computer technology (Molinari 2001), minimal contact with supervisors/support networks (Case-Smith and Mills 1996; D'Souza 2000; Mills and Millsteed 2002), and cultural variation of caseload (e.g., aboriginal clients) (Bent 1999; Minore and Boone 2002; Sheppard 2000). In addition, the literature identified the notion of the "small town" community culture as influencing confidentiality in rural practice and community's appreciation of service (Elliott-Schmidt and Strong 1995; Hegney and McCarthy 2000; Mills and Millsteed 2002).

Through interaction with clinicians practicing in northern rural and remote areas, Northern Studies Stream students are introduced to varying perspectives taken by practitioners to capitalize or offset these characteristics.

What Do You Need to Practice in a Rural Area?

Practice in rural Northwestern Ontario is characterized by geographic and professional isolation in the smaller communities, generalist as specialist practice, a dependence on the interprofessional team, and fluctuating membership of this team. These characteristics are similar to those described in the articles that examine practice in rural United States and Australia (Smith and Hays 2004; Stanton and Dunkin 2002).

The literature suggests there are clinical skills and personal characteristics necessary for success in rural practice. These include effective communication, creativity, flexibility, resourcefulness, ability to problem solve, ability to manage multiple roles (e.g., consultation versus direct intervention), computer literacy, and driving ability (Case-Smith and Wills 1996; Kohler and Mayberry 1993; Molinari 2001; Stanton and Dunkin 2002). Elliot-Schmidt and Strong (1995) conducted a survey of occupational therapists practicing in rural Australia and found that the job-related personal characteristics most often cited amongst rural therapists were flexibility, confidence, assertiveness, outgoing personality, autonomy, ability to network, lateral thinking, knowledge of community and culture, and the ability to cope with isolation and rural lifestyle. Similar personal characteristics were also found of occupational therapists practicing in the rural northwestern United States (Kohler and Mayberry 1993).

Given the importance of allowing students to assess their suitability to work in a rural setting, opportunities to introduce the students to the findings in the literature and to the experiences and perspectives of northern, rural, and remote practitioners are an important component of the Northern Studies Stream. Students are given the opportunity to discuss practice preferences, caseload management strategies, skill set, and utilization of equipment within the context of what will be successful in a rural practice setting. Students are also encouraged to consider the findings in the literature as weigh points to assess their suitability for northern, rural, remote practice.

Recruitment and Retention

Northern, rural, and remote communities throughout the world note a chronic problem in recruiting healthcare professionals (Solomon et al. 2001). In order to allow students to make informed choices, rural educators must expose them to recruitment and retention issues and to the factors that influence employment choices. Educational initiatives that promote rural practice can focus on positive elements that influence recruitment and offer solutions and strategies to overcome the perceived deterrents to choosing a rural practice. By using rural recruitment and retention indicators in the development of an education curriculum, students considering practice in a northern, rural, or remote setting will feel more prepared for the experience and may see factors they previously viewed as deterrents, as advantages.

Many personal and professional factors influence the recruitment and retention of healthcare professionals to rural and remote settings. These can be viewed as either positive or negative depending on the individual. For example, the diversity and complexity of a rural caseload may be viewed by some as an advantage and a challenge while others may view this as a stressor. Factors that influence recruitment may also influence retention but may change in priority or importance. Table 12.1 illustrates the evolution of identification of frequently cited personal positive recruitment and retention factors.

Educational programs should consider recruitment and retention research when creating informed curriculum. Inclusion of this helps students develop an understanding of the need to employ strategies to overcome anticipated challenges and to take advantage of the benefits of practice in this area.

Generalist as Specialist

Generalist as specialist practice is a hallmark of rural practice. This label describes a practice that does not fit into usual practice descriptions such as school health, rheumatology, older adult, or community mental health. The word that best captures generalist as specialist practice is "varied". Varied can refer to location, developmental stage, and/or nature of disability of the clients served.

Clinicians practicing in this way are either stimulated or taxed by the broad scope of service provision required to meet the needs of the clients. Generalist as specialist practice necessitates a breadth and depth of knowledge and skills that is facilitated by supports. These supports include a solid network of colleagues who are easily accessible for informal consultations. Educational opportunities designed to assist clinicians in maintenance of competence, despite infrequent contact with the relevant clientele, are also important support mechanisms. These supports are challenging to obtain in rural practice. Therefore, the successful generalist as specialist is one who can use technology creatively to connect with others, who embraces creative and flexible problem-solving, and who integrates the concepts of lifelong learning and reflective practice as central, essential tools for identifying needs, determining strategies, and evaluating the outcomes. Learning these strategies is a complex process that does not reliably occur as a "tack on" to a curriculum (Stanton and Dunkin 2002) and is best integrated throughout an educational program.

First Nations' Health Care Concerns as Part of Rural Practice

In many areas of the globe, First Nations' people make up a significant portion of rural inhabitants. Understanding the health care needs of First Nations' people is particularly important in Canada. While there are wide regional variations (Postl et al. 1994), it is estimated that 30–50 percent of Canadian First Nations' communities could be de-

Table 12.1. Literature scan of recruitment and retention factors. (*NSS* Northern Studies Stream)

Article (country)	Recruitment factors (listed in order of descending frequency)	Retention and/or job satisfaction factors (listed in order of descending frequency)
Polatajko and Quintyn (1986) (Canada)	Lifestyle Partner's employment Job variety Family proximity Job market Opportunity for advancement Opportunity to specialize	Lifestyle Professional freedom Variety of role Close-knit professional group Leadership opportunity Professional recognition
Beggs and Noh (1991) (Canada) (PT only)	Lifestyle	Marital status and spouse's satisfaction with lifestyle Professional tenure Career opportunity
MacIsaac et al. (2000) (Australia) (MD only)	Lifestyle Opportunity to farm Proximity to family Cheaper housing Rural upbringing	More equitable income for rural GPs Employer offered encouragement to stay
Mitka (2001) (USA) (MDs only)	Spouse employment opportunities Flexible hours Childcare availability Community factors Interpersonal skills of the recruiter (e.g., honesty and avoiding hardball sales pitches)	Article looked at recruitment only
Solomon et al. (2001) (Canada)	Leisure/recreation activities Proximity of family of origin Need for OT or PT in the area Influence of spouse/partner Incentive grant or bursary Less stressful/healthier lifestyle Lived previously in community Size of community (35.7%), possibility of working near home (31%), clinical placement as a student (24.8%), income (21.7%)	Autonomy Hours of work Variety Social camaraderie with professional peers Opportunity for personal growth Salary/benefits Accessibility with professional peers Opportunities for professional development Opportunities for involvement in OT/PT education and NSS

scribed as remote. The health and well-being of native people is dramatically lower than the general population as indicated by reduced life expectancy, increased infant mortality, increased prevalence of chronic diseases including diabetes, and greater frequency of suicide (Smylie 2001).

For indigenous people around the world, colonization has resulted in erosion of their traditional culture, marginalization, discrimination, and, consequently, ill health (Saggers 1993; Smylie 2001). By understanding the outcomes of these historical and socioeconomic patterns and the associated disenfranchisement, clinicians will be better equipped to provide an environment that is safe, supportive, and empowering to First Nations' clients.

Meeting the health care needs of these people, while ensuring respect for and preservation of their unique culture, is a challenge. Basic tenets of health promotion and illness prevention clearly recognize that the health status and health services needs of a community cannot be separated from its socioeconomic and cultural context. First Nations' people in both rural and urban centers have healthcare belief systems that may differ from the dominant population. Understanding these belief systems, developing cultural sensitivity, and adapting healthcare services to best serve indigenous people are important aspects of providing appropriate rural services.

There is also incentive to improve the quality of and the access to health care services for First Nations' people. "Basic differences between native and non-native health care providers in social structure and communication patterns are potential barriers to the effective acquisition and integration of health knowledge" (Daniel and Gamble 1995 p. 250). First Nations' people cite examples of paternalism and discrimination arising from health care workers' lack of cultural sensitivity that impede their ability to access quality medical care (Hagey 1984). Specific education is essential to ensure healthcare practitioners are efficient, effective, and competent in serving the needs of First Nations' people (Smylie 2001).

An understanding of culture, values, and belief systems for one specific culture is a foundation that may or may not be applicable to any one individual. Thoughtful clinicians must be able to value the unique nature of each individual. Developing the skills to create an understanding of and appreciation for the unique values and belief systems of each individual is the key to an effective, compassionate clinical relationship regardless of cultural background. It is conveying these nuances of the art, not the science, of practice that is the real challenge of culturally sensitive education.

Educational Initiatives for Northern, Remote, and Rural Practice

Programs which promote recruitment and preparation of practitioners for northern, rural, and remote practice in countries around the globe are well documented. These are often first established for family practice physician training and may include rehabilitation education programs as the medical programs become established. However, programs specific to rehabilitation professionals are limited. Though a variety of locations and health care practitioners have been described, the literature suggests these programs share the following characteristics:

- Fieldwork experiences that occur in rural locations to meet part or all of the fieldwork requirements of the program

- Creative strategies to accommodate for the effect of isolation on communication, including use of technology, creation of specific networks for consultations, clinical exchanges, and structured time and resources to connect

- Education about the specific sociocultural aspects of the predominant local population(s) often including the promotion of cultural sensitivity

- Discussion of specific rural practice characteristics, for example, reliance on team members, setting professional boundaries, and maintaining confidentiality in a small community

Each of these shared characteristics will be examined with selected examples provided from the literature.

Rural Fieldwork Experience

The literature suggests that those students who participate in a rural fieldwork experience are more likely to choose to practice in a rural environment (Perkins et al. 1994; Worley et al. 2000). Russell et al. (1996) examined how the attitudes and skills of occupational therapy students were influenced during a rural fieldwork experience in South Australia. Students showed a significantly positive change in attitudes toward rural occupational therapy practice in comparison to those who did not participate in this experience. Their study also suggested that students were successful in acquiring skills identified as important to rural practice.

Strategies for Coping with Isolation

Many of the programs use teleconferencing, videoconferencing, and synchronous and asynchronous use of the World Wide Web to reduce the effect of distance on satisfaction with practice (Bushy 2002). For example, in South Australia, medical interns in the rural intern training program at Flinders University spend a year in a rural setting with prescribed technologically based activities that connect the interns with the larger regional center. The interns described a higher level of confidence, greater satisfaction with on the job learning, and greater satisfaction with the clinical outcomes of their learning as a result of the experience (Mugford and Martin 2001).

Sociocultural and Rural Practice Education

Programs that successfully prepare their graduates for rural practice include a component of education that relates to the predominant population of the region (e.g., aboriginal beliefs or tropical diseases) and that describes the nature of rural practice (e.g., caseload management strategies or use of telehealth for service provision). For example, the University of British Columbia has a First Nations' House of Learning that has multiple mandates including educating the university and wider community about the concerns and issues related to First Nations' people (www.ubc.ca/longhouse). The new Northern Ontario School of Medicine plans to provide enhanced education regarding diabetes management and cardiac care given the prevalence of these issues in Northwestern Ontario.

The Northern Studies Stream as a Comprehensive Program

The Northern Studies Stream is unique in that it includes all of the shared characteristics identified as important to the education of students destined to work in a northern, rural, and remote setting. In addition, students are provided with the opportunity to complete an academic unit of study in a northern setting. It is this comprehensive approach to the preparation of clinicians that makes the program unique and innovative.

Clinical skills classes form one of the components that contribute to this thorough approach. Local clinicians are recruited to teach skills laboratories and are encouraged to share their experiences with rural practice. They emphasize the strategies they use to remain current, to meet the needs of a large, sparsely populated service area, and to maintain connections with other clinicians. These innovative strategies can be inspiring and present rural practice as an attractive alternative to urban practice. Northern Studies Stream students described this information sharing in the following way:

>> Listening to community clinicians speak about their own practices with passion and a great sense of community, made *me* feel passionate about the difference I might be able to make. I also was not aware of the opportunities that existed in rural communities until NSS. (Student PT, class of 2004)

Clinical fieldwork in rural communities is very different from that in urban centers. Students may be with a clinician who is the sole representative of his or her profession in the community and the surrounding geographical district. The student is exposed to a varied and diversely directed practice. Through observing the clinicians switching roles and incorporating strategies to maintain their expertise in a number of specialty areas, students see the creativity and flexibility of rural practice.

Rural clinicians often work in closely knit interprofessional teams that are open to maximizing the students' experience. Therefore, there is an opportunity to see the inter-reliance of rural healthcare professionals while on clinical fieldwork. Therapists often communicate with clinicians hundreds of miles away through telephone, video-conference, or email and establish a close, supportive working relationship despite never having met in person. A recent student described this phenomenon in the following manner:

>> I learned the beginnings of how to be a generalist who is innovative and flexible, using the resources/equipment that is available. I also learned how therapists of the north are resourceful, creative, problem solvers. They rely on and help each other out. (Student PT, class of 2004)

An environment where contact and support between peers can be a challenge may lead to increased worth placed on communication and feedback. Students often comment that northern, rural therapists are skilled at providing ongoing feedback.

>> While there were many changes to my understanding of rural practices probably the one theme that stands out the most is that of support. In the north, efforts were regularly made to ensure that support was accessible. There was this constant "checking in"...that does not seem to happen in larger centers...Yes, I think it's the personalities of the north combined also with the constant awareness of the risk of isolation due to the geographical elements of the north. Because of this, support was never assumed to exist and was instead continuously offered and received. (Student OT, class of 2003)

Rural people often have lifestyle and living arrangements that are new to the student on placement. Having an experienced clinician communicate with the client in a respectful and non-judging manner can be inspiring.

>> I couldn't believe how [my clinical supervisor] just walked into the most (for me) surprising/shocking circumstances with such grace. She accepted each person with such respect and non judgment and got to work setting up a relationship of trust and support. She got right down to what was important to them, what their goals were and then used the minimal resources they had in their house or their yard to set up a treatment plan. Every setting was unique and challenging. That really got me excited about a rural job. Now when I meet a challenging patient of my own I think of how she would treat them. It makes me be my best me. (Student PT, class of 2004)

Often students observe clinicians using creativity and resourcefulness to "make do" with materials and resources available, for example, bicycle inner tubes to "fix" a prosthesis or adapting a raised toilet seat to fit an all-weather outhouse.

Rural placements, in general, offer a different experience of community. Students are often surprised by the openness and inclusiveness of communities to a transient newcomer in their midst.

Native Healthcare Education

>> With the knowledge and respect of native culture and the confidence I gained from both the educational and clinical components of NSS, I approach each new client and each new situation with an open-mind, a willingness to use creativity in my assessment and treatment plans, and a greater respect for the uniqueness of each client. (Student PT, class of 2002)

Facilitating an understanding of the health care concerns of First Nations' people and strategies to facilitate culturally sensitive services is one of the priorities of the academic portion of the program. Regardless of setting it is important that healthcare students learn to explore the client's belief systems and avoid making generalizations influenced by media or historical biases. This is especially true when working with First Nations' clients and communities.

Northern Studies Stream faculty collaborate with persons from the First Nations' community to teach students how to practice accessible and effective healthcare for native clients. These native teachers make it clear that not all First Nations' people espouse traditional belief systems or values. Whether urban or rural based, First Nations' people have diverse backgrounds. Some communities have had exposure to missionaries for many generations and have developed strong religious identification as part of their community culture. They may also espouse a medical model of health beliefs similar to any other Canadian community and frown on dependence on traditional beliefs.

There are some communities that are attempting to return to traditional native ways and values to connect with their cultural past and to attempt to give meaning and direction to members struggling with alcoholism, substance abuse, suicides, and family breakdown. Having an understanding of the present realities of life for the breadth of First Nations' communities helps students avoid assumptions and stereotypes that prevent true client-centered healthcare.

Northern Studies Stream faculty and community resources have developed many teaching strategies to maximize students' understanding of effective service provision for native clients. Since the inception of the program case scenarios have been adapted to reflect the healthcare concerns of First Nations' people. Faculty rely on the wisdom of local native elders and other health care providers of aboriginal descent to create these scenarios. The scenarios are developed to help students understand the complex web of social, cultural, economic, and political determinants of health that are vital to understanding native health care challenges.

Local First Nations' experts are invited to teach native health care belief systems and priority clinical topics. For example, diabetes is a condition that has great significance to First Nations' health. Changes in traditional diet and exercise patterns have contributed to some of the highest rates of diabetes in the world among aboriginal people globally and specifically in Northwestern Ontario (Hanley et al. 1995). Increased rates of morbidity and mortality due to diabetes are at crisis levels in First Nations' communities. The students in the Northern Studies Stream spend a full week working on a community-based health scenario that focuses on diabetes in First Nations' communities.

Students have the opportunity to learn about traditional healing theories and practices from a traditional healer. These classes have taken place in several different venues including a traditional birch bark learning wigwam, a modern native health care center, and a wilderness waterfall that the students hike into with the traditional healer. At times the students have also been invited to observe and participate in spiritual ceremonies.

Students are encouraged to respect common patterns of interaction that favor a more casual conversational style of interviewing than the directive, probing questioning more common in medical interviews. Often First Nations' people may be more comfortable with silence than their "white" caregiver and less comfortable with constant eye contact. Understanding these nuances of communication style can avoid misunderstanding and allow a more comfortable exchange for both parties.

The students learn that the use of culturally familiar objects and pictures can improve the success of client education. During treatment the use of demonstration, modeling, and visual cuing is often the preferred method of learning new information or skills. For example clinicians suggest the use of a fresh moose joint from a local hunting trip to teach important concepts needed to understand arthritis.

Reflective journaling is encouraged during the Northern Studies Stream experience. Journaling provides the student with the opportunity to structure time for reflection and to receive support and encouragement to make sense of their experiences. In their reflective journals the students speak of new insights into the depth and complexity of traditional First Nations' healthcare belief systems. They are often intrigued by the union of body, mind, and spirit in the traditional health beliefs systems reflected in the teachings of the aboriginal medicine wheel. The Northern Studies Stream classes may also uncover some of the students' own preconceptions about First Nations' culture and peoples.

Concepts and strategies for providing culturally sensitive care to minority groups within a population may provide skills that can be used for many different cultural groups. One student, who is herself part of a minority group, found that she was "surprised that many of the strategies and sensitivities encouraged in caring for first nation's people would work equally as well for some of the more traditional people of my home village. I find it reassuring that people are so receptive to learning new ways of being open to other people's values and ways. I want people who care for my grandmother to keep these lessons and these attitudes in mind" (Student PT, class of 2004).

In addition to the formal academic curriculum provided during Northern Studies Stream academic units, there is an attempt to included opportunities to work with First Nations' people while on clinical placements. In some of the smaller outlying communities of Northwestern Ontario, a significant portion of the patient caseload is of First Nations' descent. Efforts are made to include a visit to First Nations' communities with the clinical supervisor as part of the clinical placement.

Innovative community connections have also been established to provide opportunities to gain further understanding of appropriate health care provision for First Nations' people. One role-emerging placement was established at a new and dynamic community health care facility that serves First Nations' people in Thunder Bay. Although they do not yet employ rehabilitation professionals the administration see this as a future priority. The student physiotherapist worked under the supervision of two First Nations' nurse practitioners while maintaining contact and supervision with a physiotherapist in a neighboring facility. The student attended all assessments of an orthopedic, neurological, or cardio-respiratory nature to offer the rehabilitation perspective. She conducted specific in-service training for other team members on assessing back, knee, and shoulder problems. She also acted in a consulting role to several community programs offered in the clinic such as creating exercise guidelines for inclusion in diabetes management teaching. Following graduation this student accepted a position working primarily with First Nations' people.

>> My experiences with both my placement at the center and Sioux Lookout and my NSS academic unit definitely consolidated my decision to work with Aboriginal peoples. It gave me confidence in my ability to work with such people. I learned about the many barriers facing Aboriginal peoples in Canada (including, stereotypical views of them from the outside world, barriers to culturally appropriate health care provision, etc). I also learned about the need to respect each individual's beliefs/cultural approach in providing health care. But, probably most of all it showed me the many rewards and joys that one receives from working with these amazing people. (Student PT, class of 2004)

Several Northern Studies Stream students have gone on to accept positions in rural communities that have a significant First Nations' population. They comment that their exposure and education on native health care have better prepared them for working effectively with their First Nations' clients.

This graduate is a member of a First Nations' community and has some unique insight into evaluating the Northern Studies Stream experience:

>> Being from a First Nations' community I recognize the need for health care providers to have some cultural understanding and sensitivity if they are to be effective in meeting the needs of my communities. Education about different cultures and immersion in different cultures are distinctly different. The first provides information that allows for ideas to surface and perspectives to be formed. The second usually alters those ideas and perspectives. [The Northern Studies Stream] introduces these concepts and instills a sense of curiosity and confidence to continue the search for understanding after graduation. (Student PT, class of 2000)

The words of these students show that they feel they have achieved an increased understanding of First Nations' healthcare concerns and some useful strategies to maximize their effectiveness when working with this population. The sentiment in the students' words suggests that these are lessons that may be implemented beyond First Nations' culture and will likely have an impact on all of the clients served by these budding clinicians.

Outcomes

Readiness for Practice Survey Results

Evaluation of the effectiveness of the Northern Studies Stream program in recruiting clinicians for northern and rural practices was conducted after ten years of the program. Surveys were sent to four graduating classes of the McMaster School of Rehabilitation Science. Respondents were asked to provide details of worksite choice and their perception of how prepared they were for rural and remote practice. The information was used to inform curricular planning and to give direction to existing recruitment and retention strategies.

A large percentage of graduates from both the Northern Studies Stream and the main campus programs reported that they felt prepared for practice in rural settings. Although the northern campus spends more time exploring rural communities and First Nations' health care as a formal part of their mandate, both groups of students increase their awareness through the use of specific northern, rural, and remote scenarios in problem-based tutorials. The inclusion of scenarios incorporating rural and First Nations' people into the mainstream curriculum may, in part, account for the feelings of preparedness for northern, rural, and remote practice expressed by the McMaster graduates.

Recruitment Outcomes

Participating in the Northern Studies Stream had a positive influence on students' choice of a rural worksite after graduation. Data collected in Northwestern Ontario through tracking surveys suggests that 11–16 percent of the participants in the combined academic and clinical experience of the Northern Studies Stream program return to Northwestern Ontario or a similar northern practice site. These northern and/or rural practice sites ranged from Northern Labrador to the southern United States. Lifestyle factors strongly affected the clinicians' choice of practice setting. The strongest motivation for choosing a northern rural or remote area to work was the small town lifestyle and recreational opportunities. Other significant factors were proximity to family and friends and a desire to return to a place similar to previous work or school locations.

According to recent graduates who had returned to work in the north, the exposure to rural practice was extremely influential on choice of employment location. The students eloquently describe the passion that has been conveyed by the clinicians about the positive aspects of practice and the strategies to overcome the challenges.

» By providing education and clinical placements in Northwestern Ontario, [the Northern Studies Stream] provides the opportunity for a number of individuals who would not otherwise consider this area, with a unique glimpse into a different reality. It replaces ignorance or assumption with knowledge and understanding. It opens minds and creates an awareness for a different way of life, challenges to practice that may never be experienced in Southern Ontario, and new and innovative strategies that clinicians use in their practices to overcome obstacles unique to northern practice. (Student PT, class of 2002)

Retention Outcomes

The Northern Studies Stream enjoys a strong level of support from local clinicians who act as preceptors, tutors, and educators. The program provides an opportunity for clinicians to remain current with the latest evidence, challenge their teaching abilities, take advantage of preceptor education opportunities, and maintain an association with a teaching university. Many local clinicians who participate in the teaching are recruited from Northern Studies Stream graduates who recognize the benefits of the program and are eager to participate in its continuance. In conversations with the Northern Studies Stream faculty, clinicians indicate that they find the opportunity to teach and supervise students contributes to their professional development and is a significant factor in their job satisfaction. As indicated by Solomon et al. (2001) these opportunities are positively linked with retention.

Conclusion

12

In our experience there are key factors that have made the Northern Studies Stream a successful, comprehensive program that prepares students for northern, rural, and remote practice. These include: strong collaborative connections with clinicians and community agencies, integration of northern, rural, and remote case studies across the curriculum, and faculty who are creative, flexible, and self-directed.

Clinicians are more likely to return to work in a northern, remote, or rural setting if they participated in the Northern Studies Stream. Those that participated in both the academic and clinical experiences were more likely to work in a northern, rural, remote setting than those who came solely for clinical fieldwork. This suggests that greater priority should be given to providing longer stay experiences which incorporate both academic and clinical education.

Lifestyle and recreation opportunities available in northern and rural communities are key factors in drawing clinicians to work in these areas. Students, as potential clinicians, should be given ample opportunity and support to explore the leisure and recreation activities that they enjoy while they are completing a fieldwork experience or an academic unit in a northern, rural, or remote community.

Educational institutions should consider promoting their health care programs in northern and rural communities to ensure that students of rural origin are strategically recruited to rehabilitation programs. These potential students are already aware of the leisure and lifestyle attributes of the north and have the added incentive to return to live near family when they graduate. Given that students of rural origin are more likely to return to work in a northern, rural, and remote community, strategic recruitment to the Northern Studies Stream should be a priority. In addition to rural origin, it may be wise to suggest to students that they will be best suited to a northern, rural, and remote experience if their personality and leisure interests match those outlined in the recruitment literature.

As this program enters its fourteenth year, future directions include: enhanced use of technology to promote connections with peers, community resources, and other faculty, design and implementation of a sustainable interprofessional component, and an enhanced appreciation of the variety of creative roles rehabilitation professionals can play within rural, remote, and/or First Nations' northern communities.

References

Beggs CE, Noh S (1991) Retention factors for physiotherapists in an underserviced area: an experience in Northern Ontario. Physiother Can 43:15–21

Bent A (1999) Allied health in central Australia: challenges and rewards in remote area practice. Aust J Physiother 45:203–212

Bushy (2002) International perspectives on rural nursing: Australia, Canada, USA. Aust J Rural Health 10:104–111

Case-Smith J, Wills K (1996) Perceptions and experiences of occupational therapists in rural schools. Am J Occup Ther 50:370–379

Daniel M, Gamble D (1995) Diabetes and Canada's aboriginal peoples: the need for primary prevention. Int J Nurs Stud 32:243–259

D'Souza R (2000) A pilot study of an educational service for rural mental health practitioners in South Australia using telemedicine. J Telemed Telecare 6:187–189

Elliot-Schmidt R, Strong J (1995) Rural occupational therapy practice: a survey of rural practice and clinical supervision in rural Queensland and Northern New South Wales. Aust J Rural Health 3:122–131

Hagey R (1984) The phenomenon, the explanations and the responses: metaphors surrounding diabetes in urban Canadian Indians. Social Sci Med 18:265–272

Hanley AJG, Harris SB, Barnie A, et al (1995) The Sandy Lake health and diabetes project: design, methods and lessons learned. Chronic Dis Can 16:149–156

Hart G, Salsberg E, Phillips D, Lishner D (2002) Rural health care providers in the United States. J Rural Health 18(suppl):211–232

Hegney D, McCarthy A (2000) Job satisfaction and nurses in rural Australia. J Nurs Admin 30:347–350

Humphreys (2000) Roles and activities of the Commonwealth Government University Departments of Rural Health. Aust J Rural Health 8:120–133

Kenny A, Ducket S (2003) Issues and innovations in nursing education: educating for rural nursing practice. J Adv Nurs 44:613–622

Kohler E, Mayberry W (1993) A comparison of practice issues among occupational therapists in the rural Northwest and the Rocky Mountain regions. Am J Occup Ther 47:731–737

MacIsaac P, Snowdon T, Thompson R, Crossland L, Veitch C (2000) General practitioners leaving rural practice in Western Victoria. Aust J Rural Health 8:68–72

Mills A, Millsteed J (2002) Retention: an unresolved workforce issue affecting rural occupational therapy services. Aust Occup Ther J 49:170–181

Minore B, Boone (2002) Realizing potential: improving interdisciplinary professional/paraprofessional health care teams in Canada's aboriginal communities through education. J Interdisciplinary Care 16:139–147

Mitka M (2001) What lures women physicians to practice in rural areas? JAMA 285:3078–3079

Molinari D (2001) Bridging time and distance: continuing education needs for rural health providers. Home Health Care Manag Pract 14:54–58

Mugford B, Martin (2001) Rural rotations for interns: a demonstration in South Australia. Aust J Rural Health 9:S27–S31

Northern Health Information Partnership (2004) An overview of health status in Northern Ontario (short report no. 2). Mary Ward, Sudbury, ON

Perkins J, Berry S, Tryssenaar J (1994) The Northern Studies stream: educating health professional in remote regions. Arctic Med Res 53:118–120

Polatajko H, Quintyn M (1986) Factors affecting occupational therapy job site selection in underserviced areas. Can J Occup Ther 53:151–158

Postl B, Irvine J, MacDonald S, Moffatt M (1994) Background paper on health of aboriginal peoples in Canada. Cited in: Bridging the gap: promoting health and healing for Aboriginal peoples in Canada. Canadian Medical Association, Ottawa

Russell M, Clark MS, Barney T (1996) Changes in attitudes and skills among occupational therapy students attending a rural fieldwork unit. Aust Occup Ther J 43:72–78

Saggers S (1993) But that was all in the past. The importance of history to contemporary Aboriginal health. Aust Occup Ther J 40:153–155

Sheppard L (2000) Work practices of rural and remote physiotherapists. Aust J Rural Health 9:85–91

Smith J, Hays R (2004) Is rural medicine a separate discipline? Aust J Rural Health 12:67–72

Smylie J (2001) A guide for health professionals working with aboriginal peoples. J Soc Obstet Gynaecol Can

Solomon P, Salvatori P, Berry S (2001) Perceptions of important retention and recruitment factors by therapists in Northwestern Ontario. J Rural Health 17:278–285

Stanton M, Dunkin J (2002) Rural case management: nursing role variation. Lippincotts Case Manag 7:48–55

Strasser RP, Hays RB, Jamien M, Carson D (2000) Is Australian rural practice changing: findings from the National Rural General Practice Study. Aust J Rural Health 8:222–226

Worley PS, Prideaux DJ, Strasser RP, Silagy CA, Magarey JA (2000) Why we should teach undergraduate medical students in rural communities. Med J Aust 172:615–617

Chapter 13

A Program Logic Model: A Specific Approach to Curriculum and Program Evaluation

13

Sue Baptiste, Lori Letts

Contents

In the current climate, evaluation as an idea and expectation is familiar to anyone who works in an academic or practice setting. We, in our roles as practitioners, are evaluated by supervisors, managers, and others to ensure quality of client care. We in turn evaluate others when asked for feedback regarding the performance of colleagues. As faculty we evaluate our students, our courses, and ourselves; and when involved in scholarly activities, evaluation is a central component of our work. The opportunity to create a new curriculum provides an opportunity to employ a conscious approach to overall evaluation. This chapter explores briefly the idea of and rationale for evaluation and illustrates the approaches taken toward evaluating our new curricula in occupational therapy and physiotherapy at McMaster University.

External Context and Expectations for Accountability

In any role within human services, there is a central ethic of accountability, more so when the institution in question resides within the public sector. In addition, it is a privilege to be engaged in the education of others, and in the preparation of individuals for specific professional practice. Such tasks, while exhilarating and fun, cannot be taken lightly. Evaluation is the manifestation of commitment and accountability to the task at hand.

The health professional climate in Ontario is one of regulation and accountability. Through the Regulated Health Professions Act of 1991 (RHPA), occupational therapists and physiotherapists (among many other professional groups) are registered to practice by professional colleges: the College of Occupational Therapists of Ontario (COTO) and the College of Physiotherapists of Ontario (CPO). Both of these colleges have developed practice competencies that must be met before graduates may practice their profession in the province (www.hprac.org/english/legislation.asp). This is the case across Canada and also in many other countries including the United States, Australia, and the United Kingdom. Entry-level competencies are derived and identified through a process of working with the professional bodies provincially and nationally, and a registration process designed. In Canadian occupational therapy, the national association, the Canadian Association of Occupational Therapy (CAOT) has developed a certification examination, successful completion of which most provinces have adopted as part of their entry to practice expectations. Canadian physiotherapists have to complete a two-part competency examination which includes a written and a clinical evaluation component. The determination of fitness to practice is complex, but the process relies upon the commitment of the colleges to work in partnership with the academic programs and professional associations. Through such relationships, it becomes clearer and easier to ensure that programs teach their students the knowledge, skills, and behaviors that are inherent within entry to practice competencies

The successful completion of a recognized accreditation process is a key responsibility of all academic programs. There may be other expectations from provincial bodies that govern education and from worldwide professional associations. Given these multiple, complex expectations it becomes evident that having a clear plan and program of evaluation of curriculum is essential as this provides an accessible and logical information bank that supports and defines program excellence. Evaluation at its broadest includes consideration of these external demands for evaluation along with internal demands such as faculty, student, and course evaluation. By bringing these together, a comprehensive approach to evaluation can be undertaken.

Internal Demands and Expectations

Faculty Evaluation

Full-time faculty members are expected to engage in a process of tenure and promotion that entails proceeding through steps from lecturer to full professor. These steps are clearly articulated and expectations are well described. In order to proceed in this manner, intensive evaluation takes place by faculty peers, students, mentors, supervisors, and self. Such evaluation encompasses reflections, observations, and ratings of faculty performance in roles, courses, and in overall academic and scholarly productivity. Therefore, it is critical that any curricular changes are undertaken with consideration of the roles and efforts that will be expended by faculty members; also, that these efforts are recognized and congruent with individual faculty member's abilities, goals, and directions.

Support for Fiscal Resources

There is also a need for evaluation data for the purpose of negotiating fiscal resources, whether this is for the maintenance of a base budget or for the determination of the "value added" by the work of the program(s) under scrutiny. A well-reasoned and developed evaluation plan with supporting data is invaluable in stating the case for excellence and continuance of an academic program.

Student Assessment/Evaluation

Student assessment is another essential element of evaluation in any curriculum. The results are reflections of the effectiveness of the overall curriculum plan. It is important that the assessment methods are congruent with the pedagogical model adopted by the program. It is also our belief that all methods of student assessment should be supported by evidence whenever possible. For example, in the earlier stages of our curricula, the occupational therapy faculty used an assessment method called a Triple Jump widely throughout the overall program (Foldevi et al. 1994; Smith 1993). A Triple Jump is a clinical reasoning exercise that uses a three-stage process providing students an opportunity to work through a clinical problem. In step 1, learners meet individually with a faculty member and are given a clinical scenario. The learner reflects on the learning issues inherent within the problem and designs a learning plan. Step 2 involves the period of time given to the learner for exploring resources and addressing the issues identified within the learning plan. At step 3, the learner returns to meet a second time with the faculty member, presenting the outcomes of the learning experience and providing a self-assessment related to the accuracy of the plan, the value of the learning, and any additional insights that are relevant. Based upon the outcomes of research into this evaluation process, the Triple Jump is now used as a formative tool and only rarely for the purposes of enhancing students' awareness of development of their clinical reasoning and critical thinking abilities.

Course Evaluation

Input from students regarding their opinions of each course is also critical. By the same token, faculty members involved in delivering each course have a similar responsibility to reflect upon their teaching experiences and provide feedback to assist in the ongoing development of the curriculum. While it is not possible or desirable to make changes in response to all feedback, receiving this input is an essential component of ongoing accountability and responsiveness to those receiving or participating in the delivery of the curriculum. Tables 13.1 and 13.2 provide examples of how course evaluation is approached in the occupational therapy and physiotherapy programs. These forms are given to students at the end of the term or at the end of the final class or evaluation session.

All student responses are collected, collated, and then run through a statistical program to provide mean and median data for use in compiling each faculty member's dossier for consideration in tenure and promotion. It is at this stage that any issues requiring remediation relative to faculty performance are identified and dealt with as appropriate. Results from course evaluations are used by course planners in making adjustments to course content and evaluations when planning the course in subsequent years.

Table 13.1. Example of unit/term and faculty evaluation used by both programs

MCMASTER UNIVERSITY MSc(PT) PROGRAM

UNIT #1
UNIT EVALUATION & FACULTY PERFORMANCE
Since all the items being rated on this form do not lend themselves to the same descriptors of quality, please use the following generic scale as a guide when you assign your ratings

1	2	3	4	5	6	7	8	9	10
Very poor	Poor			Acceptable			Good	Very good	Excellent

UNIT EVALUATION

1. Objectives (clarity, achievability)
2. Content (depth, breadth, integration across courses)
3. Organization (timetable, special events)
4. Textbooks (quality, usefulness)
5. Library resources (accessibility, quality, usefulness)
6. Human resources (accessibility, quality, usefulness)
7. Workload (balance of workload and evaluation components across courses)
8. Overall, what is your opinion of the *effectiveness* of this unit?

FACULTY PERFORMANCE

9. Organized
10. Accessible
11. Sensed problems and assisted in resolution
12. Considered/listened to student feedback
13. Flexible
14. Demonstrates professional behavior
15. Overall, what is your opinion of the effectiveness of this faculty member?

13

Table 13.2. Example of tutorial evaluation used by both programs

MCMASTER UNIVERSITY MSc(PT) PROGRAM

UNIT #1
COURSE – PROBLEM-BASED TUTORIALS
Since all the items being rated on this form do not lend themselves to the same descriptors of quality, please use the following generic scale as a guide when you assign your ratings

1	2	3	4	5	6	7	8	9	10
Very poor	Poor			Acceptable		Good		Very good	Excellent

COURSE EVALUATION

1. Objectives (clarity, achievability)
2. Organization (sequencing of events, quantity and distribution of workload)
3. Content (variety and relevance of problems, enhanced learning)
4. Evaluation (consistent with objectives, weighting of components)
5. Overall, what is your opinion of the *effectiveness* of this course?

Evaluation Elements

Basic principles of evaluation can be captured in many different ways (Patton 1989; Reisman 1994). The following rubric was developed to reflect the many facets of curriculum evaluation.

Evaluation is:

- Both science and art.

- Intended to improve program planning and delivery.

- Multifaceted: no one methodology exists. Each situation presents its own particular needs and readily interfaces with both qualitative and quantitative approaches. Objective data sources for overall program evaluation include student grades, the success rate of graduates in the credentialing examinations, and employability. Subjective data sources can include course and lecturer/faculty evaluations completed by students, student satisfaction data, plus exit and follow-up survey results.

- Participatory, involving everyone who is part of the curricular element being assessed.

- Based on rigorous standards that reflect the research process and respect existing evidence.

- Respectful of different view points and a means for debate, discussion, and reconciliation of approaches.

- Important for the continuing growth of a system or program. "Exclusive reliance on external expertise can limit an organization's ability to be clear and specific about its goals and to learn and apply lessons. Specific strategies can be built into evaluations, which are explicitly aimed at [specific] organizational characteristics" (IDRC, web/idrc.ca/en/ev).

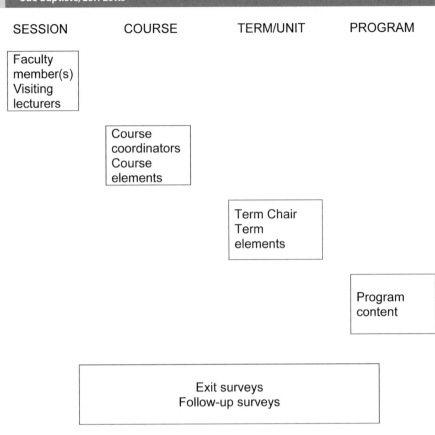

Fig. 13.1. Process of cumulative evaluation

This list of principles has been adapted from "Our Principles for Evaluation" from the International Development Research Centre (http://web/idrc.ca/en/ev) and has guided the development of our evaluation processes.

There is an important distinction between process and outcome evaluation, but both are essential to the overall evaluation of a curriculum. As stated earlier, there is a specific need to focus on evaluation in a taxonomical manner. For example, starting from the front-line of individual lectures and sessions, evaluations should progress toward collecting exit and follow-up data from graduates and alumni (see Fig. 13.1).

Evaluation Processes in Place at McMaster University

The processes for evaluating sessions, courses, terms, and units in both programs have been developed over years of experience, review, reflection, and responsiveness to change in the curriculum models as well as the expectations of learners. The processes have been framed against a backdrop of principles of problem-based and learner-centered learning. Evaluation forms that have been finalized at this stage of the entry-level masters programs are the result of many iterations over time. Indicators contained within each evaluation form (session, course, term, and faculty evaluations) are decided upon based on two key criteria: do they reflect the learning process experi-enced by the students and are they as similar as possible throughout each curriculum and both curricula when possible and appropriate? Consistency when natural and not contrived is a great help when exploring evaluative data across a process.

While both programs are invested in rigorous evaluation processes, the approaches have been different. Again, this is seen in a positive light, since by such an approach, everyone gains from insight that otherwise might be missed. For the purposes of this chapter, we are focusing on the approach taken by the occupational therapy program in engaging a program logic model (PLM) approach for overall process evaluation and for the development of a map for outcome evaluation.

Use of the Program Logic Model Approach

The PLM approach to program evaluation has been used widely in rehabilitation pro-gram development and evaluation and in designing evaluation plans within research studies (Letts and Dunal 1995; Letts et al. 1993). It has also had widespread application within the public health and social services sector (Unrau 1993). Reports of its use have shown it to be clear and useful in structuring program evaluation activities. A key characteristic of logic models is that "means" (what is done) and "ends" (the results of what is done) are separated. "Means" address the processes that are undertaken, and "ends" address the outcomes that are sought or expected. It is very easy to confuse the two and often there is no clear distinction between process and outcome. This can re-sult in a rather "muddied" picture at the end of a lot of hard work.

>> The key to a useful programme evaluation is using a systematic approach to collect reliable information about how well a programme is meeting its goals and the needs of the community. (Letts et al. 1999 p. 1)

Therefore, the adoption of a clear and concise framework from the beginning serves as an efficient manner in which to proceed with program evaluation.

Understanding the Basic Structure

The first important step in developing a PLM is understanding the basic structure. *Main components* describe the major activities of the program in one or two words. *Implementation objectives* translate those components into objectives that describe what the program is expected to do. *Outputs* are indicators of a program's implemen-tation and provide information about the delivery of services and characteristics of the people receiving the service. Outputs allow measurement of whether the program is doing what it intended to do. *Outcome objectives* relate to what is expected to change or happen resulting from the program doing what it set out to do. Although the actual measurement of the outcome objectives is not included in the model itself, each one of the outcome objectives suggests what needs to be measured thus providing a frame-work for this to be achieved. Arrows link each element of the model and clarify the re-lationships between the components (Rush and Ogborne 1991).

In our situation, all faculty members who were engaged in the curriculum planning process were familiar with the PLM approach to some degree. The Occupational Ther-apy Evidence-based Practice Research Group within the School is a collective of like-minded occupational therapy faculty colleagues who developed a workbook to help practitioners address the rather thorny question of how to evaluate programs (Letts et al. 1999). Therefore, it became a relatively simple task to activate the knowledge provided within the pages of the workbook to develop the framework we needed for moving forward in planning the curriculum evaluation for the occupational therapy program.

Developing the Model

One of the pleasures of taking the PLM approach is that it can be crafted to suit the culture and context of the agency or organization in question. The approach is generally quite flexible in terms of how to approach the task, but the foundational questions remain relatively consistent:

- What is our long-term outcome objective?
- What changes are anticipated in response to the program, i.e., short-term outcome objectives?
- What are the main components of our program?
- How can we describe the main activities through implementation objectives?
- What indicators can be used to measure the implementation objectives, i.e., outputs?
- What linkages exist between all of the components?

In order to illustrate the way we approached this task, each question will be addressed with examples given of what was developed for the McMaster Occupational Therapy Program Logic Model (Fig. 13.2).

■ **Educational Philosophy.** In order to provide a clear focus for our work, we defined our overarching educational philosophy. This one-line statement reflected our commitment to the adult learning principles of self-directed, problem-based, lifelong learning. It also declared our intention to prepare students to become reflective, entry-level practitioners who practice in a client-centered, evidence-based manner. The educational philosophy provides the beginning statement within the model while the long-term objectives are the anchor point.

■ **Long-term Outcome Objectives.** These objectives are lofty and seemingly far from reach. In fact, that is the point. These are intended to stretch the reality of today toward a better future within which these objectives can become the reality. Within these statements lies a clear link to outcome evaluation. In our case, we aimed to participate in the betterment of the health and well-being of all Canadians and graduate occupational therapy leaders and advocates for change in their profession and broad-based communities. Although it must be acknowledged that many factors beyond the educational program will influence these outcomes, their inclusion in the model reflects our belief the program can have a long-term impact to improve health of Canadians.

■ **Short-term and Intermediate Outcome Objectives.** Following the determination of the visionary focus for the curriculum, it is necessary to articulate the short-term and intermediate program objectives. These provide a bridge between the detailed levels of implementation objectives and outputs and the long-range vision. Our short-term outcome objectives were to: increase students' knowledge of core concepts needed for practice in occupational therapy; increase our students' competence with the skills needed for practice; and improve students' abilities to engage in behaviors that are appropriate to their professional role. These three objectives converge in the intermediate outcome objective of graduating entry-level occupational therapists who are competent to practice our profession in a rapidly changing health and social service context at local, national, and international levels.

At this stage our attention reverted to the top of the model in order to identify the main program components.

■ **Main Program Components.** We chose to take a longitudinal view of the program resulting in the definition of eight main components. These components reflected the process of learning experienced by the students from admission to graduation and beyond. They are:

- Admissions

- Small group tutorials/seminars

- Large group sessions

- Skills laboratories

- Independent learning

- Experiential practical (fieldwork)

- Student evaluation

- Alumni relationships

After defining the main components, we brainstormed and ultimately clarified the implementation objectives. Full details are available within the Program Logic Model (Fig. 13.2); however, highlights will be used to illustrate examples of the desired foci for this component.

■ **Implementation Objectives.** Implementation objectives should reflect the processes that are undertaken in the fulfillment of the component. For example, in the admissions component, the first step is to effectively market the program in order to attract applicants; following this, all applicants must be checked for eligibility (whether they meet the entry criteria of a four-year honors undergraduate degree or equivalent with a B average). Then, the eligible domestic candidates are interviewed, international files reviewed, and offers made in order to recruit the incoming class. Timelines should also be reflected here together with any statements that articulate underlying values; for example, as the seventh element of the admissions component we have stated clearly that we wish to ensure a heterogeneous mix of students in each incoming class. This is a very strong value of the occupational therapy faculty group, and alludes to respect and recognition of diversity.

Once the implementation objectives are identified, then the outputs follow.

■ **Outputs.** For each item within the implementation objectives, there should be corresponding output. In the case of the admissions component, outputs mirrored the ob-

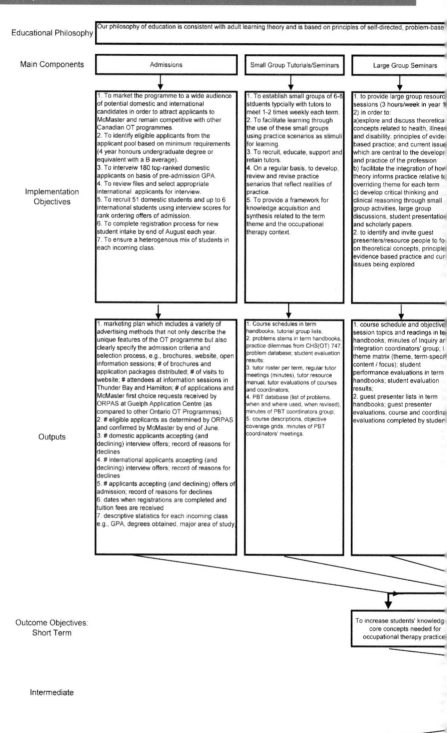

Fig. 13.2. McMaster Occupational Therapy Program Logic Model

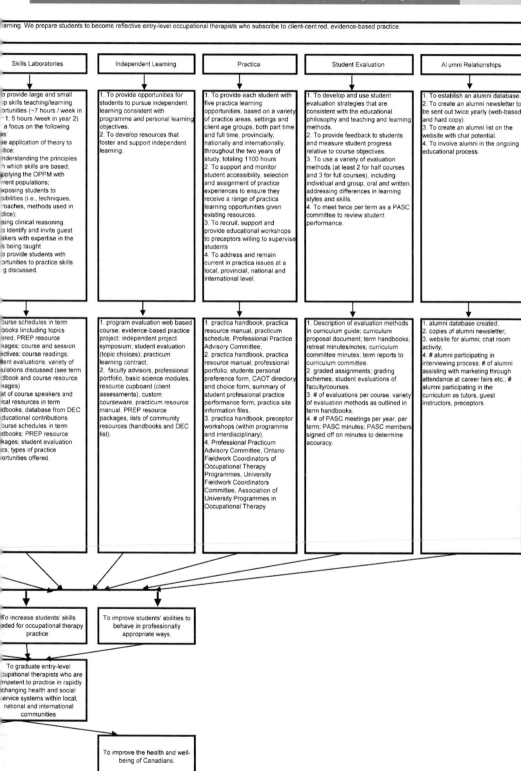

...arning. We prepare students to become reflective entry-level occupational therapists who subscribe to client-cent red, evidence-based practice.

Skills Laboratories

...o provide large and small
...p skills teaching/learning
...ortunities (~7 hours / week in
... 1; 5 hours /week in year 2)
... a focus on the following
...s:
...e application of theory to
...ctice;
...nderstanding the principles
...n which skills are based;
...pplying the OPPM with
...rent populations;
...xposing students to
...sibilities (i.e., techniques,
...roaches, methods used in
...ctice);
...sing clinical reasoning.
...o identify and invite guest
...akers with expertise in the
...s being taught
...o provide students with
...ortunities to practice skills
...g discussed.

...ourse schedules in term
...books [including topics
...ered; PREP resource
...kages; course and session
...ectives; course readings;
...ent evaluations; variety of
...ulations discussed (see term
...dbook and course resource
...kages)
...st of course speakers and
...cal resources in term
...dbooks; database from DEC
...ducational contributions.
...ourse schedules in term
...dbooks; PREP resource
...kages; student evaluation
...cs; types of practice
...ortunities offered.

Independent Learning

1. To provide opportunities for
students to pursue independent
learning consistent with
programme and personal learning
objectives.
2. To develop resources that
foster and support independent
learning.

1. program evaluation web based
course; evidence-based practice
project; independent project
symposium; student evaluation
(topic choices); practicum
learning contract;
2. faculty advisors, professional
portfolio, basic science modules,
resource cupboard (client
assessments), custom
courseware, practicum resource
manual, PREP resource
packages, lists of community
resources (handbooks and DEC
list).

Practica

1. To provide each student with
five practica learning
opportunities, based on a variety
of practice areas, settings and
client age groups, both part time
and full time, provincially,
nationally and internationally,
throughout the two years of
study, totaling 1100 hours
2. To support and monitor
student accessibility, selection
and assignment of practice
experiences to ensure they
receive a range of practica
learning opportunities given
existing resources.
3. To recruit, support and
provide educational workshops
to preceptors willing to supervise
students
4. To address and remain
current in practica issues at a
local, provincial, national and
international level.

1. practica handbook, practica
resource manual, practicum
schedule, Professional Practice
Advisory Committee,
2. practica handbook, practica
resource manual, professional
portfolio, students personal
preference form, CAOT directory
and choice form, summary of
student professional practice
performance form, practica site
information files,
3. practica handbook, preceptor
workshops (within programme
and interdisciplinary),
4. Professional Practicum
Advisory Committee, Ontario
Fieldwork Coordinators of
Occupational Therapy
Programmes, University
Fieldwork Coordinators
Committee, Association of
University Programmes in
Occupational Therapy

Student Evaluation

1. To develop and use student
evaluation strategies that are
consistent with the educational
philosophy and teaching and learning
methods.
2. To provide feedback to students
and measure student progress
relative to course objectives.
3. To use a variety of evaluation
methods (at least 2 for half courses
and 3 for full courses), including
individual and group, oral and written,
addressing differences in learning
styles and skills.
4. To meet twice per term as a PASC
committee to review student
performance.

1. Description of evaluation methods
in curriculum guide; curriculum
proposal document; term handbooks;
retreat minutes/notes; curriculum
committee minutes; term reports to
curriculum committee.
2. graded assignments; grading
schemes; student evaluations of
faculty/courses.
3. # of evaluations per course; variety
of evaluation methods as outlined in
term handbooks.
4. # of PASC meetings per year, per
term; PASC minutes; PASC members
signed off on minutes to determine
accuracy.

Alumni Relationships

1. To establish an alumni database.
2. To create an alumni newsletter to
be sent out twice yearly (web-based
and hard copy).
3. To create an alumni list on the
website with chat potential.
4. To involve alumni in the ongoing
educational process.

1. alumni database created;
2. copies of alumni newsletter;
3. website for alumni; chat room
activity;
4. # alumni participating in
interviewing process; # of alumni
assisting with marketing through
attendance at career fairs etc.; #
alumni participating in the
curriculum as tutors, guest
instructors, preceptors.

To increase students' skills
...eded for occupational therapy
practice.

To improve students' abilities to
behave in professionally
appropriate ways.

To graduate entry-level
...cupational therapists who are
...mpetent to practice in rapidly
...changing health and social
...ervice systems within local,
...national and international
communities

To improve the health and well-
being of Canadians.

Table 13.3. Example of link between implementation objectives and outputs

Implementation objective	Output
Marketing program to domestic and international applicants	Marketing plan developed with use of multiple media, e.g., website, CDROM, open information sessions
Identify eligible applicants	Number of eligible applicants confirmed by Graduate Registrar by end of June
Complete interview process	Number of domestic applicants accepting
International files reviewed	Number of international applicants; those accepting and declining
Ensure heterogeneous mix	Descriptive statistics for each class

jectives as can be seen within Table 13.3. Once the outputs are clearly defined and linked with the implementation objectives, it is time to review the overall model and determine whether it will guide the development and evaluation of the curriculum from this point onward.

■ **Linkages Between All Components.** It is also the time to determine the linkages between and among all components. In the case of our logic model, all links progress from the top to the bottom, although there is an implicit expectation that there is a feedback loop that ensures that this is an ongoing process.

Next Steps

While the focus of this section is to describe the PLM approach to curriculum evaluation, it is also necessary to comment upon the links between process and outcome evaluation of this program. At this stage, we have graduated two classes from the entry-level masters program and are poised to graduate a third. An outcome evaluation plan has been made, and some of the elements are:

- Completion of an exit survey one year post-graduation
- Analysis of outcomes in the national credentialing examination
- Survey of alumni attitudes and opinions of their professional preparation over time

Steps to complete an exit survey have been completed and results of one survey have been received. The survey is administered online one year after graduating from the program.

Conclusion

While the use of a PLM is of great assistance in organizing the development of a process evaluation curriculum plan, it does not provide information concerning the evaluations of students, faculty, courses, and sessions. It is important to go beyond applying the PLM approach to ensuring that these other essential elements are evaluated in congruence with the pedagogical approach and philosophy. Assurance of the comprehensiveness of the overall evaluation plan is reaffirmed through the process of accreditation. However, having a framework is essential to keeping curriculum development on track. The PLM is an excellent tool to which to refer once the curriculum is underway and the business of teaching and facilitating learners becomes the central task. Ensuring a systematic approach to evaluation can simplify what can become a potential confusion of data. This can also help in safeguarding from the syndrome of "evaluating for evaluation's sake"; every evaluative element should make sense according to the larger schema. Also, it is critical that the pursuit of rigorous and credible outcome evaluation is not disregarded once a model or system is put into place.

University education in Canada and elsewhere is becoming a business enterprise and, as such, requires serious commitment to public relations and a general marketing approach toward the recruitment of potential learners. This applies most specifically to professional preparation programs. Therefore, the development of a curriculum evaluation plan can provide invaluable information and data about the experience of being a student in a particular program; similarly, such data can inform all stakeholders about the quality of the graduates from that program. Accountability is a central premise and with the competitive nature of the marketplace increasing, programs that can show their commitment to excellence and their acceptance of the need for transparency will stand in good stead when students are selecting their program of choice. Similarly, such a system will provide invaluable information and input to the processes of faculty recruitment, evaluation, and promotion. As the pursuit of new knowledge is a core element of academic life, so should the application of the same principles be of equal importance in the development, support, and ongoing evolution of curricula. As the emergence of entry-level graduate programs in rehabilitation science becomes more widespread, attention to evaluation will become critical.

References

Foldevi M, Sommansson G, Trell E (1994) Problem-based medical education in general practice: experience from Linkping, Sweden. Br J Gen Pract 44:473–476

International Development Research Centre (2004) Our principles for evaluation. http://web/idrc.ca/en/ev

Letts L, Dunal L (1995) Tackling evaluation: applying a programme logic model to community rehabilitation for adults with brain injury. Can J Occup Ther 62:268–277

Letts L, Fraser B, Finlayson M, Walls J (1993) For the health of it! Occupational therapy within a health promotion framework. CAOT Publications, ACE, Toronto, ON

Letts L, Law M, Pollock N, Stewart D, Westmorland M, Philpot A, Bosch J (1999) A programme evaluation workbook for occupational therapists. CAOT Publications, ACE Ottawa, ON

Patton M (1989) A context and boundaries for theory-driven approach to validity. Eval Program Plann 12:375–377

Porteus, Sheldrick, Stewart (1997)

Reisman J (1994) A field guide to outcome-based program evaluation. Evaluation Forum, Seattle, WA

Rush B, Ogborne A (1991) Program logic models: expanding their role and structure for program planning and evaluation. Can J Program Eval 6:95–106

Smith RM (1993) The triple jump examination as an assessment tool in the problem-based medical curriculum at the University of Hawaii. Acad Med 68:366–372

Taylor, Botschner (1998)

Unrau Y (1993) A program logic model approach to conceptualizing social service programs. Can J Program Eval 8:117–134

Subject Index